AGING FEARLESSLY

A COMPREHENSIVE GUIDE TO LONGEVITY, HEALTHY
AGING, MENTAL WELLNESS, AND LIVING WITH
VITALITY AND JOY

WILLIAM J. CALLAGHAN

CONTENTS

INTRODUCTION

I remember a conversation I had with my grandmother on her 85th birthday. We sat on the porch, the sun setting behind us, painting the sky with hues of orange and pink. Looking at me twinkly, she said, "Aging is not about getting old. It's about getting wiser, learning to dance with time, and finding joy in every wrinkle." Her words struck a chord deep within me. They encapsulated a truth I had seen in my work with many older adults. The years we collect are more than just rising numbers; they are opportunities for our growth, wisdom, and laughter.

This book serves as a guide for your ongoing transformation. It is for those of you stepping into the middle and later stages of life. I wish to help you unlock vitality and wisdom, turning the aging journey into one filled with positivity and empowerment. Many view aging with much trepidation, seeing it as a "decline." But what if it could be a time of renewal and strength?

Aging can bring fears of losing independence, experiencing health issues, or facing loneliness. These are real concerns. You might worry about being unable to do what you love or feeling isolated as social circles shrink. The aim here is to address these challenges head-on. Together, we can shift the narrative from fear to resilience and joy!

The book is structured around crucial themes for a fulfilling aging experience. Physical vitality is about exercise and feeling *alive* in your body. Mental sharpness involves keeping your mind engaged and curious. Emotional well-being means nurturing your heart with kindness and compassion. Social connections are about maintaining meaningful and supportive relationships. Financial security gives you peace of mind, while spiritual growth connects you to something larger than yourself. Cultural perspectives provide a broader view, enriching your understanding of aging.

Throughout these chapters, you will find actionable strategies that you can apply in your *own* life. Real-life case studies will offer insights from those who have successfully navigated their aging journeys, and personal stories will show you the human side of these experiences. This roadmap aims to reassure you that this book is practical and insightful.

What sets this book apart is the integration of diverse cultural insights and scientific research. We will explore how different societies view aging and what we can learn from them. The stories of successful aging from around the globe will provide a broader perspective. These elements offer a unique vantage point, setting this book apart.

My background is in helping the aging population thrive. With years of experience in this field, I have seen firsthand the impact of approaching aging with a positive mindset. This book reflects my commitment to delivering guidance that is both reputable and relatable. My expertise is in this book to support and encourage you on this journey.

As I conclude this introduction, I invite you to turn the page with an open mind and heart. Embrace the opportunities that come with aging. Let us continue our life's journey together, finding joy and purpose each day.

Aging is not just an unavoidable phase but a beautiful dance with time. Let us learn the steps and move together with grace and strength.

1

EMBRACING THE JOURNEY OF AGING

As I sat with my friend Harold one crisp autumn afternoon, we watched the leaves dance to the ground, their vibrant colors showing the beauty of change. Harold, at 78, had just enrolled in an online painting class. His excitement was palpable as he shared his plans to capture the essence of each season on canvas. It struck me how this stage of life, often mislabeled as a time of "slowing down," could instead be a period of *vibrant renewal.* Harold was not just painting; he was embracing a new beginning, redefining what his golden years could be like.

THE GOLDEN YEARS: A NEW BEGINNING

Often seen as the "twilight" of life, these golden years are filled with exciting opportunities waiting to be seized. Many of us have passions and interests that have been tucked away, overshadowed by the demands of career, family, and the general busyness of life. Now is the time to dust off those dreams. If you have ever wanted to paint, write, or dive into a new field of study, this is your moment!

Online courses and community colleges offer many classes designed to inspire and educate. Whether it is learning a new language or understanding the intricacies of digital photography, the resources are abundant and waiting for your curiosity to take the lead.

Traveling, too, becomes a rich source of new experiences. Consider this the *perfect* time to explore new landscapes, meet people different from yourself, and enrich your understanding of our world.

Personal reinvention is another gift of the golden years. This stage of life offers freedom—freedom to redefine who you are and what you wish to contribute to the world.

You have spent years honing skills in a particular field. Starting a small **consultancy** or business could be the perfect way to share your expertise while keeping your mind engaged. **Mentorship** is another avenue that allows you to guide others with your accumulated wisdom. Giving back through **community service** projects can also bring profound satisfaction. **Volunteering** not only enriches the lives of others but also adds layers of meaning to your own life, creating enriching connections.

As you transition into these later years, it is natural to encounter emotional shifts. Society often imposes stereotypes about aging, painting it as a time of "decline." But such views do *not* define you.

Building self-confidence and a sense of self-worth is essential. Engage in practices that affirm your value and celebrate your achievements, no matter how small they may seem. Surround yourself with supportive voices that recognize your worth. Remember, your experiences and insights are treasures that younger generations can benefit from.

Legacy building becomes a focal point for many as they age. The stories and wisdom you have gathered over the years are invaluable. Consider writing your memoirs or a family history. These narratives can become cherished keepsakes, illuminating your journey for future generations. Creating art or projects that reflect your values is another way to leave a lasting impact.

These endeavors not only preserve your legacy but also provide a sense of fulfillment, knowing that you have imparted something meaningful and enduring to others.

Reflection Exercise: Exploring Your New Beginning

Take a moment to reflect on what you wish to explore in this stage of life. What passions have you set aside? What new interests would you like to pursue? Write these thoughts in a journal. Consider what steps you can take this week to explore one of these areas. Whether signing up for a class, planning a trip, or reaching out to volunteer, let this be the start of your new beginning.

REDEFINING SUCCESS IN YOUR THIRD ACT

As we enter the later stages of life, it is time to redefine what success truly means. For many, the traditional markers of success —wealth, career achievements, and social status—lose their shine. In their place, personal satisfaction and meaningful relationships emerge as accurate indicators of a life well-lived.

Picture a friend who found fulfillment in cultivating a community garden after retiring from a high-pressure corporate job. The accolades and financial gain did not matter anymore, but the joy of nurturing life and sharing it with neighbors *did*. This broader view of success emphasizes happiness, personal contentment, and the richness of human connections.

Setting new goals becomes a vital aspect of your redefinition. It is about aligning your ambitions with what you genuinely value *now*. Physical goals, like training for a marathon or participating in a yoga retreat, offer health benefits and create a sense of accomplishment.

These activities remind us that the body thrives on movement and challenge, no matter the age. Similarly, personal development goals, such as learning a new language or mastering a musical instrument, keep our minds engaged. Such pursuits bring a sense of achievement and joy, proving that learning is a lifelong adventure.

Reflection and self-assessment are crucial in understanding past achievements and building a foundation for future growth. Taking the time to evaluate where you have been helps illuminate your path forward.

Consider engaging in exercises that prompt you to reflect on past experiences and the lessons they taught. This introspection can be incredibly enlightening, clarifying what you want to pursue next. Journaling is a powerful tool for envisioning the future, offering a private space to explore dreams, set intentions, and chart a course for the years ahead.

Lifelong learning is a cornerstone of personal enrichment, developing our adaptability and resilience. It is not just about acquiring new skills but about keeping our sense of curiosity and engagement with the world. Enrolling in community education programs or joining online forums and discussion groups can ignite intellectual excitement. They provide opportunities to meet new people, share ideas, and stay mentally active.

Success stories abound of individuals who have embraced non-traditional paths and found profound fulfillment. Think of the former accountant who, driven by a lifelong passion for cooking, opened a small café. Or the retired teacher who began writing and published her first novel in her seventies. These are not isolated tales but real-life examples of what it means to pursue happiness over material achievements. They teach us that success is a deeply personal journey that can be reimagined and pursued at any stage of life.

As you contemplate what "success" means to you now, consider the full spectrum of your life experiences and the opportunities ahead. Embrace that your third act can be the most rewarding, filled with new adventures, deep relationships, and personal growth!

It is about crafting a life that reflects your values, desires, and dreams without the constraints of past definitions. This stage of life offers the freedom to explore and redefine success on your terms.

THE POWER OF POSITIVE AGING

The concept of "positive aging" is grounded in the belief that our attitudes toward growing older can profoundly influence our health and well-being. Positive aging suggests that we can enhance our mental and physical health by embracing this stage of life with optimism and enthusiasm.

Scientific studies underscore this, revealing that individuals with a positive outlook on aging tend to live longer, healthier lives. A study involving over 14,000 adults found that those satisfied with their aging process were significantly less likely to suffer from chronic diseases and had a lower mortality risk. This is not merely about avoiding illness; it is about thriving.

Personal anecdotes offer vivid illustrations. Consider Jane, a lively 82-year-old who sees each wrinkle as a story, each gray hair as a sign of wisdom earned. Her zest for life is infectious, and she often attributes her vitality to her positive perspective, which she maintains through daily gratitude and mindfulness practices.

Maintaining such positivity in the face of aging challenges will require intentional strategies. One practical approach is cultivating gratitude. This can be as simple as noting three daily things you are thankful for. By focusing on the good, you create a buffer against negativity.

Mindfulness and meditation also play crucial roles. These practices teach us to live in the moment, reducing the stress and anxiety accompanying aging. They encourage a calm mind and a peaceful heart, helping you to appreciate the present without the weight of past regrets or future worries. Mindfulness exercises, even for a few minutes daily, will significantly elevate your mood and outlook.

The role of community and support networks cannot be overstated. As social creatures, our connections with others profoundly affect our quality of life. Joining social clubs or groups with shared interests provides opportunities to meet new people and forge meaningful friendships. Whether it is a book club, a gardening group, or a choir, these interactions can enrich your life with shared experiences and laughter.

Building intergenerational relationships is equally rewarding. Spending time with younger family members or youth in your community can offer fresh perspectives and invigorating energy. These bonds foster a sense of belonging and purpose, reminding us that we are valued and needed.

Society often perpetuates misconceptions about aging, which can lead to negative stereotypes and self-doubt. We can challenge these myths, particularly those surrounding memory loss and cognitive decline. While it is true that some cognitive changes occur with age, they are not as dire or inevitable as often portrayed. Many older adults maintain sharp minds well into advanced age.

Highlighting stories from various cultures can counteract these myths. For instance, in regions where elders are revered and active in community life, such as in Okinawa, Japan, aging is *celebrated*, not *feared*. These communities demonstrate that aging can be a period of continued growth and contribution with the right mindset and environment.

Reflection Section: Cultivating Positivity

Take a moment to reflect on your daily routine. How often do you practice gratitude? Consider starting a gratitude journal. Write down a few things each day that bring you joy or contentment. Notice how this simple act shifts your perspective over time.

Also, explore mindfulness techniques that resonate with you. A short morning meditation or an evening reflection can become part of your routine. These practices, though small, can profoundly impact your view of aging, turning each day into 24 hours, supporting positivity and fulfillment.

CULTIVATING A GROWTH MINDSET FOR LATER LIFE

As we grow older, our mindset plays a pivotal role in facing and adapting to changes and challenges. Carol Dweck's research on growth mindset highlights the belief that abilities and intelligence can develop with effort and learning. This perspective is not just for the young; it also holds profound implications for older adults.

This attitude empowers you to see aging as a time ripe with possibilities. A growth mindset opens your heart and mind to personal development and adaptability, encouraging you to face new experiences with curiosity and enthusiasm. Embracing this mindset can significantly enhance your life satisfaction, as demonstrated by many older adults who have transformed their lives by heartily welcoming inevitable change.

Consider the story of Margaret, a 70-year-old who decided to learn digital photography. Initially daunted by technology, she shifted her perspective by seeing the challenges as growth opportunities. Margaret's journey symbolizes how adopting a growth mindset can open doors previously thought closed.

This mindset is about overcoming obstacles and seeing hurdles as stepping stones to new adventures. By cultivating such a mindset, you tap into a reservoir of potential that can lead to newfound passions and a deeply fulfilling life.

To foster a growth mindset, start with practical exercises that help reframe limiting beliefs. Identify thoughts that hold you back, such as "I'm too old to learn this," and replace them with empowering alternatives like "I can learn new things at *any* age."

Setting realistic yet challenging goals also aids in this shift. Aim for objectives that push you *slightly* beyond your comfort zone. Achieving these goals fosters a sense of accomplishment and fuels further growth. The transformation may be gradual, but each step forward reinforces the belief that growth is possible, no matter what your age.

Adaptability and flexibility are intrinsic to a growth mindset. Embracing change enhances opportunities and satisfaction in life. Whether adapting to modern technologies or embracing shifts in social roles, flexibility allows you to navigate life's unpredictability with grace.

Imagine attending a family gathering and using a video call platform to connect with distant relatives. It might feel strange at first, but the joy of bridging distances makes it very worthwhile. Similarly, as social roles evolve, embracing new responsibilities (or letting go of past ones) can lead to personal enrichment and deeper relationships.

Continuous personal development underlies a growth mindset. Engaging in creative pursuits like making art or playing music stimulates the mind and nurtures the soul. Participating in workshops and seminars offers avenues for this growth and skill-building. These activities keep the mind sharp and give you a sense of purpose and achievement.

Fostering a growth mindset means not merely adapting to aging but thriving within it. Each new skill and challenge overcome adds to your reservoir of wisdom and experience. It is about embracing life with curiosity and a willingness to evolve.

The world is vast, with endless opportunities to learn and grow. By cultivating a mindset open to new experiences, you will enrich your life with depth and meaning.

2

PHYSICAL VITALITY AND LONGEVITY

I recall when my neighbor, a spry 76-year-old named Ruth, challenged me to walk briskly through our neighborhood park. As we strolled, she shared her secret to maintaining energy and vitality: regular movement. Ruth's practice of daily walks, occasional swims, and light gardening kept her active and engaged. Her story illustrates a vital truth: movement is not just an *activity but* a form of medicine that nourishes our bodies and spirits.

Physical vitality is *essential* for a fulfilling life and can transform how we experience our later years.

MOVEMENT AS MEDICINE: TAILORED EXERCISES FOR AGING BODIES

Exercise plays a fundamental role in managing and preventing many age-related health issues. Studies have shown that regular physical activity, even in moderate amounts, can significantly reduce the risk of chronic diseases such as heart disease, diabetes, and certain cancers. Regular exercise can improve sleep quality, enhance mood, and lower anxiety.

You might find exercise daunting, especially if your mobility is limited. However, exercise does not have to mean running marathons or lifting heavy weights. It can be as simple as walking daily, stretching, or swimming. These activities are gentle on the joints and immensely benefit your overall health.

Individuals like Ruth, who have embraced exercise as a part of their daily routine, share stories of transformative health improvements. Many find that incorporating regular movement helps them feel more energetic and capable. For instance, **swimming** is an excellent low-impact exercise that supports cardiovascular health without putting undue stress on the joints. Similarly, **cycling**, whether outdoors or on a stationary bike, offers a fantastic way to improve endurance and maintain muscle tone. **Strength training**, using resistance bands or light weights, can help build muscle mass, which is crucial for maintaining balance and preventing falls.

Consistency is vital to reap the full benefits of exercise. Establishing and sticking to a routine can lead to significant health improvements over time. Creating a weekly exercise plan with various activities can keep things exciting and ensure that different muscle groups are worked. Setting achievable fitness goals, such as **walking** for 30 minutes daily or attending a **yoga** class twice a week, can provide motivation and a sense of accomplishment.

It is essential to listen to your body, adjust your routine to prevent injury, and ensure that exercise remains enjoyable!

Motivation can sometimes wane, especially when faced with obstacles such as inclement weather or a busy schedule. One effective strategy is to find an exercise friend or join a group. Having someone to share the experience with can make exercise much more enjoyable and provide accountability.

Additionally, technology offers various tools to help you stay on track. Fitness apps can track your progress, set reminders, and even connect you with virtual communities for support and encouragement. These tools turn exercise into a social activity, making it more friendly, engaging, and less of a solitary task.

Reflection Section: Building Your Exercise Routine

Consider starting with small, manageable kinds of movement to build your exercise routine. Reflect on your activities: dancing, walking, or gentle stretching. Write down a few exercises you would like to try this week. Think about how you can incorporate them into your daily life.

Could you take a short walk in the morning or evening? Perhaps join a local class or group that interests you? By taking these steps, you can create a routine that keeps you active and enhances your overall well-being.

NUTRITION FOR LONGEVITY: BEYOND THE BASICS

Imagine sitting down to a vibrant plate of food, each bite delicious and packed with nutrients that fuel your body and may add years to your life. This is the power of nutrition in promoting longevity.

A balanced diet impacts every part of your health, from your heart to your brain.

Antioxidants are crucial in reducing inflammation, a silent contributor to many chronic diseases. These potent compounds are found in colorful fruits and vegetables, like berries and leafy greens, which can help protect your cells from damage.

Meanwhile, omega-3 fatty acids found abundantly in fatty fish like salmon are vital for maintaining heart health and supporting brain function. They help reduce inflammation and are linked to lower risks of heart disease and cognitive decline.

Going beyond the basics, there are advanced nutritional concepts that can further enhance your health.

Intermittent fasting, for example, is not just about *when* you eat but how it can promote cellular repair and boost your metabolism. Giving your body regular breaks from digesting food allows it to focus on healing and maintenance.

Probiotics, the beneficial bacteria found in fermented foods like yogurt and sauerkraut, are another powerful tool. They support gut health, which is increasingly recognized as a cornerstone of overall well-being. A healthy gut can improve digestion, enhance your immune system, and affect your mood.

Incorporating longevity-promoting foods into your daily meals does not have to be complicated. Starting your day with a **breakfast** rich in fiber and protein can set a positive tone. Consider oatmeal topped with a handful of berries and a sprinkle of chia seeds rich in omega-3s. For **lunch,** a salad filled with dark leafy greens, various colorful vegetables, and a serving of grilled salmon can provide essential nutrients. **Dinner** might include a hearty vegetable soup, stir-fry with tofu, or lean chicken seasoned with turmeric—a spice known for its anti-inflammatory properties. **Snack** wisely by choosing nuts packed with healthy fats or a small bowl of Greek yogurt for a protein boost.

Let us address some common nutritional myths that are often confusing.

One such myth is that older adults do not need as much protein as younger people. Maintaining muscle mass as you age is vital;

adequate protein intake supports this. Aim to include a source of protein in each meal, whether plant-based or animal-based.

Another misconception is that supplements can replace a varied diet. While supplements can be helpful, especially if you have specific deficiencies, they should not be relied upon as a substitute for eating a wide range of whole foods. Always consult your healthcare provider before starting any new supplement regimen to ensure it complements your dietary needs.

As we explore nutrition, remember that it is more than just eating. It is about nourishing your body and savoring the flavors of life. By making thoughtful food choices, you can boost your vitality and enjoy the many benefits of a healthy lifestyle.

MASTERING MOBILITY: TECHNIQUES FOR JOINT HEALTH

Joint health is vital for keeping mobile and ensuring a superior quality of life as we age. Our joints bear the weight of our daily activities, and over time, the wear and tear can lead to conditions like arthritis. This common issue affects many people, causing pain and stiffness that can limit movement. Arthritis is not just an inconvenience; it can impact your ability to perform simple tasks and enjoy activities you love. Maintaining a healthy weight is crucial in reducing the strain on your joints. Excess weight can exacerbate joint problems, increasing the risk of pain and inflammation.

By focusing on joint health, you can prevent mobility issues and continue to lead an active, independent life.

Consider incorporating specific exercises and techniques to support and improve joint function. Stretching is an excellent way to maintain flexibility and ensure joints remain lubricated. Simple routines, like morning **stretches** or gentle **yoga** poses, help keep your joints supple and ready for the day. **Strengthening exercises** are equally important, as they build the muscles around your joints, providing additional support and reducing the likelihood of injury. You do not need heavy weights; even light resistance bands can make a difference.

These exercises can help you stay mobile and active, reducing the risk of falls and injuries from weakened muscles and stiff joints.

Lifestyle changes play a significant role in protecting and preserving joint health.

Proper footwear is essential. Shoes that offer good support can help maintain correct posture and reduce joint stress. When your feet are well-supported, your knees, hips, and back are less likely to suffer from strain. Additionally, being mindful of your posture can prevent undue joint stress. Simple adjustments, like sitting up straight or using ergonomic chairs, can significantly impact.

Modifying activities to suit your physical condition is an innovative idea. For instance, if kneeling becomes difficult, consider using a kneeling pad or a gardening bench to reduce stress on your knees while doing outdoor chores.

Exploring medical and non-medical interventions can relieve joint pain and inflammation. Over-the-counter anti-inflammatory medications are often recommended to manage pain and swelling. However, it is essential to consult with your healthcare provider to ensure these medications are suitable for you.

Alternative treatments, such as acupuncture and massage therapy, have gained popularity for their potential to alleviate joint pain. Acupuncture, which involves inserting thin needles into specific points on the body, can help reduce pain and improve joint function. Massage therapy can relieve muscles by relaxing, improving circulation, and easing joint tension.

Reflection Section: Enhancing Joint Health

Consider how you can integrate these joint health strategies into your daily life. Reflect on your current routine and identify areas that might benefit from change. Could you add a few minutes of stretching each morning? Perhaps invest in a pair of supportive shoes or a posture-friendly chair? Write down a few actionable steps this week to support your joint health.

These minor changes can lead to significant improvements, helping you maintain mobility and enjoy a more active lifestyle.

EMBRACING ALTERNATIVE THERAPIES: YOGA AND TAI CHI

In your mind, picture the sun gently warming your skin as you stand barefoot on the grass, moving deliberately and gracefully. This is the essence of practicing yoga and tai chi—which offer many benefits for both body and mind, particularly as we age.

These forms of exercise are more than just movement; they are practices that enhance balance, coordination, and mental clarity. You engage muscles, build strength, and improve flexibility with each pose and movement. Also, time spent on these practices offers a sanctuary for the mind, reducing stress and promoting peace and clarity.

Yoga and tai chi are particularly suited for older adults because they are gentle yet powerful. They encourage you to connect with your body, to move at your own pace, and to honor your limits—while gently pushing them.

For those new to yoga, simple poses like Cat-Cow and Child's Pose can help introduce the body to movement and stretching. These poses gently open joints and muscles, relieving tension and stiffness.

On the other hand, Tai chi involves a sequence of slow, deliberate movements, often described as "meditation in motion." Beginners might start with simple movements, focusing on maintaining balance and flow. Both practices improve coordination and help prevent falls, a key benefit as balance declines with age.

The mind-body connection is a central theme in yoga and tai chi. These practices are about more than physical exercise; they integrate health's mental and spiritual aspects.

Mindful breathing is a fundamental technique for calming the mind and reducing stress. This practice encourages you to focus on the rhythm of your breath, allowing each inhale and exhale to guide your movements and thoughts.

Meditation is often incorporated into these sessions, promoting more profound relaxation and mental clarity. You may find a greater connection between your mind and body through regular practice, leading to improved overall well-being and a more centered outlook on life.

Understanding the cultural and historical roots of yoga and tai chi can enhance your appreciation for these practices.

In ancient India, **yoga** has evolved over thousands of years, blending physical postures with meditation and spiritual insight. Its comprehensive approach to health has made it a global phenomenon, embraced by people of all ages and backgrounds.

Tai chi, rooted in Chinese martial arts, has been practiced for centuries. It emphasizes gentle, flowing movements that harmonize the body's energy, or "qi." In Chinese culture, tai chi is a physical exercise and a way to cultivate balance and tranquility, both physically and spiritually.

These practices offer a rich tapestry of benefits, enhancing physical vitality while nurturing mental and emotional health. Whether you are drawn to the fluid movements of tai chi or the meditative poses of yoga, both provide valuable tools for maintaining health and balance. They invite you to explore your capabilities, find joy in movement, and connect with a tradition that has sustained countless individuals throughout history.

As you incorporate these practices into your life, you may discover a newfound sense of vitality and inner calm, enriching your daily experiences and supporting your journey through the years.

Participating in exercises like yoga and tai chi enhances physical health and develops a deeper connection to yourself and the world around you. These practices provide a foundation for sustained well-being, allowing one to age with strength and serenity.

This chapter has explored the role of movement in inspiring and maintaining vitality. Next, we will delve into the importance of mental sharpness, providing strategies to keep your mind active and engaged as you explore the richness of your later life.

3

MENTAL SHARPNESS AND COGNITIVE HEALTH

I remember visiting my uncle George, who was well into his eighties, and I was marveling at how sharp his mind remained. Whenever we spoke, he dazzled me with his stories and the clarity he recalled past events. One day, I asked him how he managed to keep his mind so vibrant. With a knowing smile, he said, "It's all about the fuel you give your brain. Feed it right, and it will serve you well."

His words encapsulated a simple truth: what we eat profoundly impacts our cognitive health. Understanding this connection is crucial as we seek to maintain mental sharpness throughout our lives.

Diet plays a pivotal role in cognitive performance, influencing everything from memory to problem-solving abilities. Omega-3 fatty acids in fishlike salmon and mackerel, are vital for maintaining synaptic plasticity, learning, and memory. They enhance neurotransmitter functions and help improve blood flow to the brain, making them a critical component of a brain-healthy diet.

Antioxidant-rich foods, such as berries and dark chocolate, also contribute significantly. These foods combat oxidative stress, which can damage brain cells, by neutralizing free radicals and promoting overall brain health. They are more than delicious treats; they are potent allies in preserving cognitive functions as we age.

Incorporating specific brain-boosting foods into your diet can make a noticeable difference in cognitive health. Leafy greens like spinach and kale are rich in vitamins and minerals that support brain function. They provide essential nutrients that protect against cognitive decline, helping to keep your mind agile and responsive. Nuts and seeds, particularly those high in vitamin E, offer another layer of protection. Vitamin E is known for its neuroprotective properties, which can help delay the onset of cognitive decline.

Including these foods in your daily meals gives your brain the nutrients to stay sharp and focused.

Supplements can also play a supportive role in cognitive enhancement. Ginkgo biloba, a popular herbal supplement, is renowned for improving blood flow to the brain. This increased circulation can enhance cognitive functions, particularly memory and concentration. B vitamins are equally essential, as they are involved in energy production and neurotransmitter synthesis, both critical for maintaining mental clarity and focus. While supplements can be beneficial, consulting with a healthcare provider is essential to ensure they are appropriate for your health needs.

For practical dietary integration, consider starting your day with a smoothie packed with brain-healthy ingredients: Blend spinach, berries, a handful of nuts, and a splash of almond milk for a refreshing and nutritious start.

Lunchtime salads can include a variety of greens, seeds, and a sprinkle of olive oil, which is rich in antioxidants.

For dinner, incorporate oily fish, like salmon, and a side of steamed vegetables to provide a balanced and brain-boosting meal.

These simple changes can significantly impact your cognitive wellness, offering sustained energy and mental clarity throughout the day.

Reflection Section: Creating a Brain-Healthy Menu

Take a moment to reflect on your current eating habits. Are there opportunities to incorporate more brain-boosting foods into your diet? Consider planning a week's worth of meals that include these nutritious options. Write down a few ideas for each meal, ensuring variety and balance. This exercise helps you plan and encourages mindfulness about what you consume, supporting your cognitive health.

MENTAL FITNESS: COGNITIVE EXERCISES TO STAY SHARP

Following the path of mental fitness is like a workout for your brain, keeping it agile and resilient as the years go by. Just as physical exercise strengthens the body, mental exercises fortify the mind. This concept of mental fitness is rooted in **neuroplasticity,** which refers to the brain's incredible ability to reorganize itself by forming new neural connections throughout life. Neuroplasticity does not fade with age; it remains vital to maintaining cognitive health.

You can stimulate these connections by engaging in activities that challenge the brain, keeping your mind sharp and flexible.

Cognitive engagement acts like a mental agility course, honing your ability to think clearly, solve problems—and stay creative.

There are countless ways to give your brain the exercise it craves. Puzzles and brainteasers, such as Sudoku or crosswords, are excellent for stimulating different brain areas. These games encourage logical thinking and problem-solving, providing a delightful way to strengthen your mental faculties.

Learning a new skill or language is another powerful method. It requires your brain to work harder, forming new connections and pathways. Whether picking up a musical instrument or mastering a new language, these activities challenge your brain in exciting and beneficial ways. The satisfaction of conquering a complex puzzle or communicating in a new tongue will prove your brain's adaptability and strength.

Regular mental workouts can significantly slow the progression of memory loss and cognitive decline. Keeping your brain engaged creates a buffer against the natural aging process. Cognitive exercises enhance problem-solving skills, allowing you to approach challenges with creativity and confidence.

They also boost your thinking ability, improving your processing and retaining information. Consistence in these activities is vital. Much like physical exercise, the benefits of mental fitness accumulate over time, leading to a more robust and resilient mind. These exercises are not just about *preserving* what you have; they are about *enhancing* your cognitive abilities, giving you the tools to navigate life's complexities easily.

Set aside dedicated time each day for cognitive exercises. It could be a few minutes in the morning or a leisurely afternoon session. The important thing is to make it a *habit.* Many apps and online platforms are designed to help you train your brain. These tools offer a variety of games and challenges tailored to different skill levels, making it easy to find something that suits you that you enjoy.

Integrating these exercises into your life ensures that your brain remains an active and vibrant part of your ongoing experience.

Reflection Section: Building Your Mental Fitness Routine

Consider creating a weekly plan that includes different cognitive activities. Write a schedule incorporating puzzles, language learning, or other brain-engaging tasks you enjoy. Think about how you can vary these activities to keep things interesting. This plan helps you stay organized and encourages you to explore new ways to challenge your mind.

As you engage in these exercises, notice how your mental clarity improves and your confidence in tackling everyday tasks.

MINDFULNESS PRACTICES FOR MENTAL CLARITY

Start your day with a few quiet moments, your mind as calm as a gentle stream. **Mindfulness,** a practice rooted in ancient traditions, can bring peace and clarity to your everyday life. It centers on being present, allowing you to focus on what is happening without judgment.

This focus on the present helps to reduce stress, which is often a silent thief of mental clarity. Mindfulness can enhance your concentration and mental well-being, creating a foundation for a healthier mind.

One of the simplest ways to incorporate mindfulness into your routine is through meditation. This practice involves sitting quietly and focusing on your breathing or a particular thought. It allows the mind to settle and the body to relax.

As you breathe deeply, stress levels decrease, and your mind becomes more precise. Another technique is focused breathing. Concentrating solely on your breath can quieten the constant chatter of the mind, bringing you into a state of calmness and focus. These practices can be tailored to fit into any part of your day, providing moments of tranquility and clarity amidst the hubbub of life.

There are many mindfulness techniques to explore, each offering unique benefits. **Guided meditation** sessions can help you relax and unwind, providing a structured approach to meditation. These sessions often involve listening to a soothing voice guiding you through the process, allowing you to focus inward.

On the other hand, body scan techniques involve mentally scanning your body from head to toe, noticing areas of tension, and consciously relaxing them. This practice enhances your awareness of bodily sensations and helps you connect with yourself more deeply.

Both techniques are accessible and adaptable, allowing you to choose what resonates most with you.

Mindfulness offers significant cognitive benefits, supported by research. Regular mindfulness practice has been shown to decrease symptoms of anxiety and depression, which can cloud mental clarity and hinder daily functioning. By reducing these symptoms, mindfulness creates a more positive mental environment, allowing your brain to function optimally.

Additionally, mindfulness enhances memory retention and recall. Being present trains your brain to focus better, improving your ability to remember details and information.

These cognitive benefits underscore the power of mindfulness as a tool for maintaining your mental sharpness.

Incorporating mindfulness into daily activities can be straightforward. Consider taking a mindful walk in nature. As you walk, pay attention to the sensations in your body and the sights, sounds, and smells around you. This practice grounds you in the present and connects you to the natural world, enhancing your peace and clarity.

Creating a peaceful meditation space at home can also support your mindfulness practice. Choose a quiet corner, add a comfortable chair or cushion, and perhaps a few calming elements like candles or soft music. This space becomes a retreat where you can practice mindfulness regularly, reinforcing the positive effects on your mental clarity.

Mindfulness is more than just a practice; it is a way of life that can profoundly impact how you experience the world. Integrating mindfulness into your routine nurtures cognitive health and enhances overall well-being.

As you explore these practices, you will find more balance, focus, and joy in your daily life.

UNDERSTANDING AND COMBATING COGNITIVE DECLINE

As we grow older, it is natural for changes to occur in our brain's structure and function. These changes can influence how we process information, recall memories, and perform everyday tasks. While some degree of cognitive decline is a normal part of aging, it is essential to recognize the early signs and the contributing factors.

The brain, like any other organ, ages over time, and this can lead to gradual shifts in mental acuity. You might notice moments of forgetfulness, such as misplacement of keys or struggling to find the right word. Occasional confusion or difficulty concentrating can also occur. These unsettling signs are not definitive indicators of *significant* cognitive decline. Instead, they remind us to pay closer attention to our mental health—and take proactive steps to maintain it.

There are several strategies you can adopt to combat cognitive decline and keep your mind sharp:

Engaging in regular physical activity is one of the most effective methods. Exercise increases blood flow to the brain, delivering essential nutrients and oxygen that support brain health. Walking, swimming, or cycling can profoundly impact your cognitive well-being, keeping your brain alert.

In addition to physical activity, nurturing your social connections is crucial. Staying socially active stimulates cognitive engagement, providing opportunities for conversation, laughter, and shared experiences. Whether joining a book club, volunteering, or simply spending time with friends and family, these interactions enrich your mental life and help protect against cognitive decline.

Creating a supportive environment at home can further enhance cognitive health. Organizing your living spaces to reduce clutter and stress can make a significant difference. A tidy, well-arranged home promotes focus and tranquility, allowing your mind to function more efficiently. By establishing routines and keeping your environment orderly, you create a space that supports mental clarity and reduces the likelihood of cognitive slip-ups.

Consider using memory aids and organizational tools, such as calendars, reminder notes, or digital apps, to help keep track of appointments and tasks. These tools can ease the mental load, allowing you to focus on what is essential.

Many resources are available to support individuals experiencing cognitive decline, including medical interventions and community support.

Cognitive therapies and rehabilitation programs are designed to enhance mental function and compensate for areas of difficulty. These therapies focus on strengthening memory, attention, and problem-solving skills, offering tangible improvements in daily life.

Additionally, support groups provide a sense of community and understanding, offering a platform to share experiences and learn from others facing similar challenges. Caregivers can benefit from these resources, gaining insights and strategies to support their loved ones effectively. It is essential to seek professional advice when considering medical treatments or interventions, ensuring they align with your needs and circumstances.

As we explore these aspects of cognitive health, remember that *proactive* measures can significantly impact your mental well-being. You can maintain your cognitive vitality and enjoy a fulfilling life by staying active, connected, and organized.

These strategies combat cognitive decline and enhance your overall quality of life, allowing you to engage with the world meaningfully. Embrace these opportunities to nurture your mind and continue exploring the richness of life with confidence and curiosity.

As we have seen in this book, aging is about maintaining what you have and discovering *new* ways to thrive and grow.

4

EMOTIONAL WELL-BEING AND RESILIENCE

When I think about emotional well-being, I am reminded of my dear friend, Clara, who always radiated a serene calm despite numerous significant challenges. She had an uncanny ability to navigate life's difficulties gracefully, attributing much of her resilience to her emotional intelligence.

Clara's presence was proof of how emotional intelligence (EQ) can enhance our lives, especially as we age. EQ is the ability to understand and manage our emotions while recognizing the feelings of others. It plays a crucial role in forming better relationships, making sound decisions, and maintaining overall mental health. Unlike IQ, which measures cognitive abilities, EQ focuses on our life's emotional and social parts. These aspects become increasingly significant as we age, helping us adapt to change and connect with others.

Emotional intelligence comprises several key components: self-awareness, self-regulation, motivation, empathy, and social skills.

- Self-awareness involves recognizing your emotions and understanding how they affect your thoughts and behavior. It is the first step toward emotional intelligence, allowing you to identify your feelings and their impact.
- Self-regulation is about controlling your emotions and impulses, ensuring you respond to situations thoughtfully rather than impulsively.
- Motivation is using your emotions to stay focused on your goals, even when challenges arise.
- Empathy, a cornerstone of EQ, is the ability to understand and share the feelings of others, fostering deeper connections and understanding.
- Finally, social skills involve managing relationships and building networks, essential for effective communication and collaboration.

Enhancing self-awareness is a vital step toward improving your EQ. Journaling is an excellent tool for gaining emotional clarity. Writing down your thoughts and feelings creates a space to process your emotions and reflect on your reactions. This practice can help you identify patterns in your behavior, providing insights into how you respond to different situations.

Mindfulness practices, such as meditation or deep breathing exercises, can also increase present-moment awareness. These techniques encourage you to focus on the here and now, reducing distractions and allowing you to connect with your emotions more intensely.

Empathy plays a significant role in aging, as it helps us build deeper connections and improve our relationships. As we grow older, the ability to empathize becomes even more important, allowing us to relate to others and understand their perspectives. Active listening is a powerful technique for developing empathy.

By giving your full attention to the speaker and acknowledging their feelings, you foster an environment of trust and understanding.

Perspective-taking exercises, where you imagine yourself in another person's situation, can also enhance your empathy. These practices improve your relationships and enrich your interactions, making them more meaningful and rewarding.

Regulating emotions effectively is crucial for maintaining emotional well-being, especially during stress or conflict. Breathing exercises can be a simple yet powerful way to manage your feelings. By taking slow, deep breaths, you activate the body's relaxation response, helping to calm your mind and reduce stress.

Cognitive reframing is another technique that can help you change negative thought patterns. It involves challenging and altering unhelpful thoughts, allowing you to view situations more positively and balanced. By practicing these methods, you can develop greater emotional control, enabling you to respond to life's challenges with resilience and composure.

Reflection Exercise: Enhancing Your EQ

Consider setting aside time each day to reflect on your emotions. Start a journal where you can jot down your thoughts and feelings. Notice the emotions that arise and how they influence your reactions. Try incorporating mindfulness practices into your routine to increase present-moment awareness.

Engage in active listening during conversations, and practice empathy by putting yourself in others' shoes. As you explore these practices, observe how your emotional intelligence evolves and how it enriches your relationships and, thus, your overall well-being.

THE HEALING POWER OF GRATITUDE AND REFLECTION

In emotional well-being, gratitude is a transformative power that often goes unnoticed. At the end of a long day, reflect on moments that bring a smile or warmth to your heart. This simple act of acknowledging the good can *significantly* enhance your emotional health. Studies have shown that cultivating gratitude can lead to increased happiness and reduced symptoms of depression.

When we focus on what we *have* rather than what we *lack*, we shift our perspective from scarcity to abundance. This change in outlook reduces stress and improves our relationships, as gratitude fosters appreciation and positivity. Personal stories abound of individuals who have found new joy and purpose through gratitude, illustrating their profound impact on life.

Incorporating gratitude into your daily life does not require any grand gestures. Simple practices can bring about substantial change. Gratitude journaling is one such technique. Setting aside a few minutes daily to write about things you are thankful for creates the habit of recognizing and celebrating the positives.

Specific prompts can guide you, such as listing three things you appreciate about your day or recalling a recent act of kindness. Additionally, daily gratitude rituals can reinforce this mindset. Expressing thanks for the good things in your life at the end of the day by saying them aloud or sharing them with a loved one will make the day positive. These practices anchor us in the present, reminding us of the beauty even in the simplest moments.

Reflection, much like gratitude, is another powerful tool for personal growth. Reflecting on life experiences allows us to gain deeper self-understanding and resilience. Looking back on our journey, we can identify patterns, recognize growth, and learn from past decisions.

Creating a timeline of significant life events can help visualize your progress and milestones. This exercise provides clarity, showing how each experience in your life has contributed to who you are today. Reflective questions can further guide introspection, prompting you to consider what lessons you have learned and how they have shaped your path.

Emotional healing often finds its roots in reflection. By revisiting past experiences, you can process emotions and foster healing.

Writing letters to past selves is a therapeutic way to address unresolved feelings or acknowledge personal growth. These letters allow you to communicate with earlier versions of yourself, offering compassion, forgiveness, or encouragement.

Engaging in guided reflection sessions with a therapist or coach can also provide support. These sessions create a safe space for exploring emotions and gaining new perspectives. Reflection lets you release lingering pain and embrace a more balanced emotional state.

Reflection Exercise: Gratitude and Life Review

Take a moment to try gratitude journaling. Write down three things you are grateful for today. Allow yourself to savor these moments, no matter how small.

Next, create a simple timeline of crucial life events. Reflect on how each event has influenced your path. Consider writing a letter to your past self, expressing what you have learned and how far you have come. Use these exercises to deepen your understanding of yourself and cultivate a mindset of gratitude and reflection.

BUILDING EMOTIONAL RESILIENCE: OVERCOMING SETBACKS

Emotional resilience is the inner strength that allows you to adapt to life's challenges and recover from setbacks. It is a vital quality that enables you to face adversity with courage, maintaining your mental health and well-being even when the going gets tough.

Resilient individuals share specific characteristics, such as optimism, flexibility, and perseverance. They can remain calm under pressure and use their experiences as steppingstones for growth.

Developing resilience becomes increasingly important as we age, helping us navigate life's inevitable difficulties with grace and determination.

Building resilience is not about *avoiding* difficulties but learning how to *respond* constructively. One effective strategy is cultivating a staunch support network of friends and family who can offer guidance and encouragement when needed. These relationships provide a safety net, offering emotional sustenance during challenging times.

Practicing problem-solving skills and adaptability also strengthens resilience. When faced with a problem, try breaking it down into manageable parts and brainstorming viable solutions. By approaching challenges with a flexible mindset, you will adapt to new circumstances and find ways to thrive truly.

The mindset you adopt plays a significant role in your resilience. Reframing challenges as opportunities for growth can transform how you perceive and respond to them. Instead of viewing a setback as a failure, see it as a good learning experience leading to personal development.

This shift in perspective can foster a more positive outlook, enabling you to tackle obstacles with renewed vigor. Affirmations can further reinforce this mindset. Regularly reminding yourself of your strengths and capabilities builds confidence and prepares you to face *whatever* life throws.

Real-life examples of resilience are all around us. Consider the story of Mary, who found solace and purpose in volunteering at the local community center after losing her life partner. Through helping others, she not only healed her wounds but also discovered a fresh sense of fulfillment.

Then there's Daniel, who overcame a serious illness by focusing on rehabilitation and setting small, achievable goals. His health journey taught him the value of patience and determination.

These personal accounts illustrate that resilience is not about avoiding adversity but embracing it as a catalyst for transformation.

Each person's path to resilience is unique, shaped by their experiences and challenges. Some find strength through community support, drawing on the collective wisdom and encouragement of those around them. Others turn inward, using reflective practices such as meditation or journaling to process emotions and gain clarity. Regardless of the approach, the common thread is a willingness to confront challenges with an open heart and mind. This openness allows you to adapt, learn, and grow, building a reservoir of strength that supports you through life's trials.

Resilience is a lifelong endeavor cultivated through practice, reflection, and a willingness to embrace change. It is about recognizing that setbacks are not the end but a necessary part of life. By nurturing resilience, you equip yourself with the tools to face adversity with courage and grace, turning challenges into opportunities for growth and renewal. As you continue this path, remember that resilience is not about *perfection* but *progress*— finding strength in yourself and those around you.

FINDING JOY AND PURPOSE IN EVERYDAY MOMENTS

As we move into the later stages of life, the quest for joy and purpose often takes center stage. Finding meaning in daily activities is not just an idle pursuit but a vital component of emotional well-being. This search for purpose offers psychological benefits that resonate deeply, enhancing our overall quality of life. When we have a sense of purpose, we feel more connected to ourselves and the world around us. It anchors us, giving us a reason to get up each morning with enthusiasm and a sense of direction.

On the other hand, joy brings light to our days, enriching even the simplest of moments. This combination of purpose and joy creates a fulfilling life, regardless of age.

To cultivate joy, you might consider engaging in creative hobbies. Activities like painting or playing a musical instrument can unlock a sense of wonder and accomplishment. These pursuits allow you to express yourself, providing an outlet for creativity that can be therapeutic and invigorating. You do not need to be a professional artist or musician; creating can bring immense satisfaction.

Practicing random acts of kindness is another way to invite joy into your life. Helping others, whether through volunteering or making small gestures like writing a thoughtful note, can uplift your spirits and create a ripple effect of positivity.

Mindfulness offers a pathway to greater appreciation and enjoyment of life. By being fully present, you savor each experience, noticing the details that might go unnoticed. Mindful eating, for instance, encourages you to appreciate your food's flavors, textures, and aromas. This practice transforms meals into sensory experiences, grounding you in the present moment.

Similarly, techniques for appreciating the beauty in everyday surroundings can heighten your awareness of the world around you. Whether it is the vibrant colors of a sunset or the gentle rustle of leaves in the trees, taking the time to notice details like that can enhance your sense of joy and connection to life.

Discovering your purpose can be a transformative experience. This involves identifying what truly matters to you and aligning your actions with those values. Setting intentions that reflect your values can guide you toward a more purposeful life. These intentions act as a compass, directing your efforts and energy toward meaningful pursuits.

Volunteering or mentoring are excellent ways to contribute to your community and find purpose. By sharing your skills and wisdom, you not only enrich the lives of others but also find fulfillment in knowing that your contributions make a significant difference.

As we explore these themes, we must recognize that joy and purpose are not destinations or end points but ongoing inclusions in your life. They require attention and intention, inviting us to live with curiosity and gratitude. By embracing these practices, you can create a life of meaning and happiness, nurturing your emotional well-being and enriching your daily experiences. Joy and purpose are within your reach, waiting to be discovered and savored each moment.

As this chapter ends, consider how these insights will lead you toward a more vibrant and fulfilling existence. With these foundations, you are well-prepared to explore the next chapter, which focuses on social connections and community engagement.

5

SOCIAL CONNECTIONS AND COMMUNITY ENGAGEMENT

I remember when my neighbor, Ellen, shared her experience moving to a new city following her retirement. Initially, she felt lost amid unfamiliar streets and faces. But Ellen, with her characteristic warmth, decided to host a small gathering. She invited neighbors for tea and conversation, slowly turning strangers into friends. Her story highlights the profound impact of social connections, which are crucial for health and happiness.

Strong relationships are not just pleasant but vital for longevity and mental well-being. Studies, such as those by Amit A. Shah, M.D., have shown that social interactions enhance cognitive flexibility more effectively than brain games. Loneliness, on the other hand, poses risks akin to obesity and smoking, leading to depression and anxiety. Just as Ellen found joy and support in her new community, maintaining and building connections will profoundly enrich our lives as we age.

The art of staying connected involves both initiating and nurturing relationships. Making new friends might seem daunting initially, but joining clubs or groups that align with your interests can lead to opportunities. Whether it is a book club, a gardening group, or a walking club, shared interests provide a natural foundation for building relationships.

Regular catchups with friends or family, whether in person or through phone or video calls, help to maintain these bonds. These interactions do not have to be lengthy or elaborate; even short, meaningful conversations can keep connections strong. Scheduling these interactions as part of your routine will ensure they happen, much like Ellen's tea gatherings, which became a cherished tradition in her neighborhood.

Technology offers powerful tools for maintaining social connections, especially when physical distance is a barrier. Social media platforms like Facebook and Instagram allow you to stay in touch with distant friends and family, easily sharing moments and updates. Online communities and forums can also provide a sense of belonging and engagement. They connect you with others who share your interests, offering spaces for discussion and support.

As highlighted in a review of digital technology's impact, mobile technology enhances social well-being by connecting you to family and healthcare resources. Engaging with these platforms can combat isolation, providing companionship and information at your fingertips.

Despite the many ways to connect, barriers such as social anxiety or geographical distance can make building relationships quite challenging. Improving conversation skills can help overcome these obstacles, allowing you to engage more comfortably with others. Simple techniques like active listening and asking open-ended questions can make interactions more enjoyable and meaningful. Organizing local meetups or gatherings can also bring people together, creating opportunities for face-to-face interactions. These gatherings do not have to be large or formal; even small potlucks or coffee mornings can foster community and togetherness. Creating these moments of connection helps to bridge gaps, bringing people close despite the distances that might otherwise keep them apart.

Reflection Section: Exploring Social Connections

Consider taking a moment to reflect on your current social connections. Are there opportunities to strengthen existing relationships or form new ones? Write down a few activities or groups that interest you, and think about how you can get involved. Is there someone you have not spoken to in a while? Perhaps schedule a call or send a message. These small steps can lead to meaningful interactions, enhancing your social life and overall well-being.

COMMUNITY AND BELONGING: FINDING YOUR TRIBE

Imagine a bustling community center on a weekday morning, filled with the lively chatter of people participating in various activities. This is where individuals come together to attend events and find a sense of belonging and purpose. Being part of a community offers more than just companionship; it provides emotional resilience and a framework of support that enhances life.

Engaging with a community can uplift your spirits, offering a sense of purpose that adds meaning to each day. It is about "finding your tribe," those individuals who share your values and interests, creating a network of support that contributes to your well-being.

Identifying and joining communities that resonate with you can take some time and exploration. Local community centers and libraries are excellent starting points. They often host various activities, from art classes to discussion groups, designed to unite people. Attending these events can open doors to new friendships and connections.

Similarly, workshops and local fairs provide opportunities to meet like-minded individuals. These fun gatherings are fertile ground for building relationships based on shared interests. By stepping into these spaces, you can discover groups that align with your passions, enriching your life with new experiences and connections.

Participating in group activities is a powerful way to strengthen bonds and create lasting friendships. Shared experiences, whether in a book club or a group fitness class, help forge meaningful and enduring connections. These activities offer a common ground where conversations flow naturally, fostering camaraderie and mutual respect.

Being part of a discussion group can ignite intellectual curiosity while joining a sports team or exercise class can enhance physical *and* social health. These interactions create shared memories and experiences, building a community where you feel valued and understood.

Nurturing a sense of belonging within your community requires your active involvement. Volunteering for local events or initiatives is a beautiful way to contribute and make a difference. It allows you to engage with others while supporting causes that matter to you, fostering a deeper connection to your community.

Taking on leadership roles in clubs or organizations can also enhance your sense of belonging. By stepping into these roles, you can shape the community's direction and influence positive change. These contributions enrich the community and provide personal growth and fulfillment for you, reinforcing your place within the group.

Reflection Section: Discovering Your Community

Reflect on your current involvement in community activities. Are there groups or events that interest you but have yet to explore? Consider visiting a local community center or library to discover what is available. Write down a few activities that align with your interests and consider how you might get involved. Whether it is attending a workshop or volunteering for an event, such steps can help you *find your tribe* and build meaningful connections!

VOLUNTEERING AND GIVING BACK: CREATING IMPACT

Volunteering can transform lives, both for those who give *and* those who receive. It offers a profound sense of purpose, enriching your days with meaning and connection to the world. As you volunteer, you contribute to your community and enhance *your* well-being. Research highlights the mental health benefits of volunteering, showing that it can reduce feelings of loneliness and depression.

When you help others, your focus shifts from personal worries to the community's needs, offering a refreshing perspective on life. Many volunteers share stories of fulfillment and joy found through their service, illustrating how even small acts of kindness can create significant ripples of positivity.

Finding the right volunteering opportunity is about aligning your passions with the needs of your community. Start by identifying organizations that reflect your values and interests, such as animal welfare, environmental conservation, or education. Look for roles matching your skills and availability, ensuring your contributions are meaningful and sustainable.

If mobility is a concern, consider virtual volunteering options. Many organizations offer remote roles like mentoring, tutoring, or administrative support, allowing you to contribute from home. The key is to choose opportunities that excite you and fit seamlessly into your life, making volunteering an enriching and enjoyable experience.

Volunteering also opens doors to new friendships and professional connections. You naturally build relationships with fellow volunteers and organization staff as you work alongside others. These connections can lead to lasting friendships, offering companionship and support beyond the volunteer setting. Volunteering provides opportunities to collaborate on community projects, allowing you to expand your network and learn from others' experiences.

Engaging with a diverse group enriches your social life and broadens your horizons, fostering a sense of belonging and community. These connections often extend beyond the volunteer role, enhancing your personal and professional life.

Giving back also fosters personal growth, offering opportunities to develop new skills and gain insights into community needs. Volunteering can help cultivate leadership and organizational skills as you take on responsibilities and coordinate with others. It encourages you to step out of your comfort zone, fostering adaptability and resilience.

Through volunteering, you gain a deeper understanding of the challenges faced by your community and the impact of collective action. This awareness enriches your perspective, inspiring you to continue making a difference. The skills and experience gained through volunteering can also enhance your confidence, empowering you to contribute in new and meaningful ways.

Reflection Section: Finding Your Volunteer Path

Take a moment to reflect on your interests and values. Consider organizations or causes that resonate with you. Write down a few volunteering opportunities and consider how you might get involved. Whether virtual or in-person, local or global, find a role that aligns with your passions and strengthens your connection to the community.

NAVIGATING FAMILY DYNAMICS: STRENGTHENING BONDS

Family relationships are unique in our lives, *particularly* as we age. Strong family ties provide a foundation of emotional support, enhancing our quality of life in significant ways. These bonds offer comfort and companionship, forming a safety net that can catch us during times of need.

Intergenerational relationships, where different age groups within a family engage and learn from each other, are especially beneficial. They offer a unique perspective, allowing wisdom to flow between generations. Grandparents often find immense joy and purpose in teaching their grandchildren, while the young bring fresh energy and a new outlook on life. This mutual exchange enriches the lives of *everyone* involved, fostering a sense of continuity and belonging.

Yet, maintaining these connections requires effort and understanding. Open communication is the cornerstone of healthy family relationships. It is essential to create an environment where everyone feels heard and respected. Active listening is a powerful tool in this regard. You gain a deeper understanding of their perspectives by genuinely focusing on what family members say without interrupting or judging.

This practice builds trust and empathy, paving the way for more meaningful interactions. Regular family meetings or check-ins can also facilitate open dialogue. These gatherings provide opportunities to discuss concerns, share updates, and strengthen connections. They do not have to be formal; even a casual dinner or a Sunday brunch can serve as a platform for honest conversation.

Family dynamics often shift as we age, presenting new challenges and opportunities. Roles within the family may change, with independence sometimes giving way to the need for support from younger generations. Balancing this shift can be delicate, as it involves maintaining autonomy while accepting needed help.

Communicating openly about these changes and expressing needs and expectations is essential. Navigating the transition from *caregiver* to *care recipient* can also be challenging. It requires patience, understanding, and a willingness to adapt to new circumstances. These transitions can bring families closer, fostering deeper connections and mutual respect.

Creating family traditions can strengthen these bonds and create lasting memories. Traditions offer a sense of identity and continuity, connecting family members across generations. Planning annual family reunions or gatherings can be an excellent way to celebrate these connections. These events provide opportunities for family members to reconnect, share stories, and create new memories.

Shared hobbies or interests can also form the basis of family traditions. Whether it is a weekly game night, a holiday baking session, or a summer camping trip, these activities unite family members, reinforcing bonds and creating cherished moments.

As we conclude this chapter, remember that family relationships are vital to our lives. They offer support, love, and a sense of belonging that enriches our aging experience. By nurturing these bonds, we create a foundation of emotional resilience that supports us through life's various challenges and joys.

6

FINANCIAL SECURITY AND PEACE OF MIND

I remember a conversation with my father at the kitchen table, where he shared his meticulous approach to managing finances after retirement. A retired schoolteacher, he had always been disciplined with money, but retirement introduced new challenges. With a cup of coffee, he explained how he mapped out every expense, from groceries to medical bills, ensuring that each dollar had a purpose. His commitment to smart budgeting gave him peace of mind, allowing him to enjoy his retirement years without financial stress.

This approach is not just about numbers but about creating a comfortable and secure lifestyle where financial worries do not overshadow your (well-deserved) rest.

Creating a detailed budget is the cornerstone of financial security in retirement. It involves understanding both current and future expenses and planning accordingly. The budget often comprises essential living costs, such as housing and healthcare. It is crucial to account for these expenses first, ensuring your basic needs are met.

Housing costs might include mortgage payments or rent, utilities, and maintenance. Healthcare, particularly as we age, requires careful consideration—factor in insurance premiums, prescription medications, and potential out-of-pocket costs.

Once these essentials are covered, you can allocate funds for discretionary spending, including travel, hobbies, and leisure activities that bring you joy and fulfillment.

Effective budget management is essential to maintain financial stability. Budgeting apps or software will simplify this process, offering modern solutions for tracking income and spending patterns. With the rise in technology usage among older adults, these tools have become increasingly accessible. Apps like YNAB (You Need a Budget) and EveryDollar focus on helping users make informed spending decisions, providing a clear picture of where their money goes each month. Setting up automatic payments for recurring bills can prevent missed payments and late fees, ensuring your budget stays on track.

These strategies help you manage your finances efficiently, freeing up mental space for more enjoyable pursuits!

Regular budget reviews are essential to staying aligned with your financial goals. Quarterly budget assessments allow you to evaluate your spending and make necessary adjustments. This practice keeps your budget dynamic, responding to changes in your lifestyle or circumstances. For instance, if you notice an increase in healthcare costs, you might need to adjust other budget areas to accommodate these changes.

Inflation can also impact the cost of living, necessitating periodic reviews to ensure your budget remains realistic. By taking the time to reassess your financial situation, you maintain control over your resources, adapting to life's inevitable fluctuations.

Maximizing retirement income requires careful management and strategic investments. Exploring part-time work or consulting opportunities can supplement your income, providing additional financial security. Many retirees find that engaging in work they *enjoy* boosts their finances and enriches their lives! Evaluating the benefits of annuities or pension plans can offer a steady income stream, ensuring that your financial needs are consistently met. Annuities, for example, can provide a reliable income source, helping you manage expenses without depleting your savings. Understanding these options and how they fit into your financial plan is crucial for long-term security and peace of mind.

Reflection Section: Creating Your Budget

Take the first step towards financial peace by creating a detailed budget. List your essential expenses, including housing, healthcare, and discretionary spending like travel and hobbies. Consider using a budgeting app to track your income and expenses. Schedule regular reviews to ensure your budget remains aligned with your goals.

This exercise helps you manage your finances and provides a clear roadmap for a secure and comfortable retirement.

FINANCIAL PLANNING FOR UNEXPECTED EXPENSES

Having an emergency fund is like having a safety net that can catch you when life's trapeze wobbles a bit. That dedicated savings account stands between you and the stress of unforeseen expenses, giving you peace of mind.

Imagine this fund as a financial cushion, softening the blow of sudden costs like medical emergencies or urgent home repairs. But how much should you save? This varies depending on your financial situation. A good rule of thumb is to aim for one to two years' worth of living expenses, enough to cover what is not handled by guaranteed income like Social Security. This might sound daunting, but setting a specific target helps guide your savings efforts and clarifies your financial goals.

Building and maintaining an emergency fund requires commitment and strategy. Start by setting aside a small percentage of your monthly income. Even a modest amount of consistent contribution will grow over time. Consider those occasional windfalls, like tax returns or bonuses, as opportunities to boost your funds. Treating these extras not as spending money but as a chance to fortify your financial safety net strengthens your ability to handle life's surprises without derailing your financial plans.

This approach builds your savings and fosters your financial discipline, helping you prioritize long-term security over short-term gratification.

Insurance options can further enhance your financial security, safeguarding against significant economic risks. Health insurance is necessary, especially in retirement, where medical expenses can quickly accumulate. Evaluating plans that offer comprehensive coverage is crucial in ensuring you are protected against high medical costs.

Long-term care insurance is another consideration. It covers services not typically covered by regular health insurance, such as assistance with daily activities, should the need arise. This coverage can offer financial relief and preserve your assets for other needs. Understanding these insurance options and how they fit into your financial plan adds a layer of protection for yourself and your loved ones.

Managing debt during retirement is equally essential for financial peace. High-interest debts can drain your resources, making it difficult to save for emergencies. Prioritizing these debts for faster repayment is a wise strategy. It reduces the overall interest paid and frees up funds that can be redirected toward more productive uses, like your emergency fund.

Debt consolidation is another option to explore. This involves combining multiple debts into a single loan with a lower interest rate, simplifying payments, and potentially reducing your monthly financial burden. These strategies help you regain control over your finances and pave the way for a more secure and stress-free retirement.

Reflection Section: Building Your Emergency Fund

Think about your current financial situation and identify how much you might need in an emergency fund. Write down an achievable monthly savings goal and consider any windfalls you could allocate to this fund. Reflect on your insurance coverage and debt management strategies and determine if adjustments are necessary to bolster your financial security.

Taking these steps helps ensure you can face unexpected expenses confidently and competently.

SIMPLE STRATEGIES FOR FINANCIAL INDEPENDENCE

Achieving financial independence in retirement means reaching a point where your financial resources allow you to live comfortably *without* relying on external assistance. It is about having the freedom to pursue interests and passions without financial constraints dictating your choices.

Imagine waking up each day knowing that your finances are secure enough to allow you to travel, take up a new hobby, or spend more time with the family without the stress of financial limitations. This type of independence offers peace of mind, allowing you to focus on what truly matters—exploring new interests or spending time with loved ones. This level of freedom and security is empowering and enriches the quality of your retirement years.

To achieve this financial freedom, diversifying your income streams is vital. Rather than relying solely on one source, such as a pension or Social Security, consider exploring various investment opportunities. Investments can range from stocks and bonds to real estate and mutual funds. Each has risks and rewards, so choosing options that align with your comfort level and financial goals is crucial.

Diversifying your portfolio helps mitigate risk, as different assets often perform differently under the same economic conditions. By spreading your investments across several streams, you increase the likelihood of maintaining a steady income, even if one area falters. This strategy supports financial independence and provides a good safety net, ensuring you have multiple sources to support your lifestyle.

Reducing unnecessary expenses is another effective strategy to bolster savings. Often, small, habitual spending can add up over time without us realizing it! Take a closer look at your monthly expenses and identify areas where you can cut back. This could include dining out less frequently, reviewing subscription services, or finding more affordable alternatives for entertainment.

By consciously reducing non-essential spending, you will free up funds that can be redirected towards savings or investments.

Passive income is critical in achieving financial independence, providing income streams that require minimal ongoing effort. Real estate investments, for example, can generate rental income, offering a reliable cash flow each month. While managing properties does involve some work, it can be outsourced to property management companies if preferred.

Another avenue for passive income is investing in dividend-paying stocks or bonds. These investments provide regular income through dividends or interest, supplementing your primary income sources.

Incorporating passive income into your financial plan creates a robust foundation for maintaining your lifestyle without needing *active* work. This diversification supports financial independence and contributes to a more balanced and secure financial future.

Obtaining financial literacy is an ongoing process, essential for making informed decisions that support your financial independence. Staying educated about financial matters empowers you to navigate the complexities of retirement planning confidently.

Consider attending financial education workshops or seminars offering valuable insights and up-to-date information on various economic topics. Reading books or articles on personal finance and investing can also enhance your understanding, providing practical advice and strategies to apply to your financial plan.

By continually expanding your financial knowledge, you equip yourself with the tools you need to adapt to changes in the economic landscape, ensuring your financial independence remains intact.

UNDERSTANDING AND ACCESSING AVAILABLE RESOURCES

Finding your way in the maze of government programs and benefits can feel daunting, but these resources are vital for ensuring financial security in retirement. Social Security, a source of retirement income for many, offers a safety net based on your work history.

Understanding eligibility criteria is crucial. To qualify, it would be best to have worked and paid into the system for at least 10 years. The age at which you start receiving benefits can affect the amount you receive, with the full retirement age varying based on the year you were born. Medicare and Medicaid are equally important, providing essential healthcare services.

Medicare, primarily for those sixty-five and older, covers hospital stays, doctor visits, and some home health care. Medicaid assists with medical costs for those with limited income and resources. Knowing what each program offers and how to access them can significantly ease the financial burdens associated with healthcare in retirement.

Community resources and support systems extend *beyond* government programs, offering additional assistance layers. Senior centers often serve as hubs for free financial counseling, helping you understand the complexities of retirement planning. They guide budgeting, investing, and managing assets, ensuring you make informed financial decisions.

Charitable organizations, many of which focus specifically on seniors' needs, offer essential services ranging from food assistance to utility support. These organizations are crucial in filling gaps and addressing needs that government programs might not fully cover. Connecting with these local resources can provide invaluable support, helping you to maintain a stable and secure financial profile.

Applying for financial aid requires careful preparation and organization. Gathering the necessary documentation is a fundamental step. This might include proof of income, identification, and relevant financial records. Having these documents organized and readily available can streamline the application process, reducing stress and increasing the likelihood of approval.

Seeking assistance from financial advisors or social workers can also be beneficial. These professionals are well-versed in navigating the system and can offer guidance on completing applications accurately and efficiently. Their expertise can make a significant difference, ensuring you access the benefits and resources you are entitled to.

Proactive resource management is vital to optimizing available programs and benefits. Scheduling annual reviews of your benefits and programs lets you stay informed about any changes that might affect your eligibility or the level of support you receive. These reviews allow you to reassess your financial situation and adjust matters as needed, ensuring you continue effectively meeting your needs.

Community workshops offer ongoing learning opportunities, keeping you updated on untapped resources and strategies for managing your finances. Engaging in these workshops enhances your knowledge and connects you with others working out similar issues, providing a sense of community and shared purpose.

As we explore these resources, it is essential to remember that they are tools designed to *support* you in achieving financial security and peace of mind. Understanding and accessing these programs and benefits lays a solid foundation for a stable and fulfilling retirement.

This chapter aims to equip you with the insight and confidence to come to a good understanding of the complexities of financial planning, ensuring that you can enjoy your golden years without the weight of economic uncertainty.

As we move forward, consider how these strategies can enhance your financial well-being and empower you to live the life you envision.

CHANGING OUR RELATIONSHIP
WITH AGING

"Aging is just another word for living."

— CINDY JOSEPH

There is a lot of fear about aging. We spend our younger days longing to be grown up, and as soon as we are out of our twenties, we start to dread every birthday, every reminder that we are getting older. We notice the wrinkles, gray hairs, and differences in our bodies, and society conveys that this is all bad. One of the first things we discussed here was the power of positive aging, and as you will see much later in this book, this is something they get right in the "Blue Zones," where people live long and healthy lives. As you will see, a lot of that has to do with lifestyle, but it also has a lot to do with attitude.

Much as we fear aging, we all want to live well *for as long* as possible. We cannot do that without aging, so our relationship with it needs to change. We need to see our later years as a valuable part of the whole story of our lives, not something to fear or as something that marks the end of what we once knew. I hope that by the end of this book, you'll have a clear idea of what you can do to support your health and well-being as you get older, and I hope you'll come to view this next chapter of your life as a time you can enjoy! I want to help as many people as I can to get to the same understanding, and it is for this reason that I have interrupted our reading journey here: I would like to ask for your help...

To connect this book with the readers looking for this kind of guidance, I will need reviews—and by taking just a few minutes to write one, you can help me reach even more people.

Leaving a review of this book on Amazon will make it easy for new readers to find it and ensure they set off on a mission: *age fearlessly.*

Reviews make it easier for people to find the guidance they seek, so a few words from you could make an enormous difference. Wouldn't it be wonderful if fewer people feared aging and knew precisely what they could do to look forward to good health, vitality, and joy in their later years? I believe that if we work together, we can make that happen.

Thank you so much for your support! You are making a real difference to others.

7

SPIRITUAL GROWTH AND INNER PEACE

I n the quiet stillness of the early morning, while the world still slumbers, I find solace in a simple ritual that has become my soul's sanctuary. Sitting comfortably in my favorite armchair, I close my eyes and allow my breath to guide me into a calm state. This practice, known as meditation, serves as a doorway to spiritual growth and inner peace.

For many, meditation is a powerful tool that nurtures the spirit and inspires a sense of awakening. It helps us connect with ourselves deeper, offering clarity and tranquility amid the chaos of everyday 21st-century life. Meditation is not about escaping reality but engaging with it more *fully*, allowing us to explore the depths of our consciousness and discover the profound peace within.

There are various forms of meditation, each offering unique pathways to spiritual insight. Transcendental meditation, for instance, involves silently repeating a mantra, a specific word, or a sound to settle the mind into restful alertness. This practice promotes inner silence and deep relaxation, dissolving stress and enhancing awareness.

Guided meditation, on the other hand, involves listening to a gentle voice that leads you through a visualization or narrative, focusing the mind and encouraging relaxation. These forms of meditation provide emotional balance by calming the mind and reducing anxiety, allowing us to reflect on our lives with greater compassion and understanding.

Starting the practice of meditation may seem challenging, but it need not be complicated. Begin with setting aside a few minutes daily in a quiet space where you feel comfortable. Creating a peaceful meditation space can enhance your practice, offering a dedicated area that invites serenity. You might add a cushion or chair, soft lighting, and calming elements like candles or gentle music.

For beginners, focused breathing exercises are an excellent way to start. Sit comfortably, close your eyes, and pay attention to your breath. Notice the sensation of the air entering and leaving your body. If your mind wanders, gently guide your focus back to your breath. Over time, this practice can deepen your connection to yourself and provide a lovely sense of spiritual grounding.

Mindfulness, closely related to meditation, plays a significant role in enhancing spiritual well-being. It involves being fully present in the moment and aware of your thoughts, feelings, and surroundings without judgment. Mindful walking, for example, transforms a simple walk into a meditative experience by encouraging you to focus on each step, the sensations in your body, and the environment around you. This practice fosters a deeper awareness of the present moment, helping you appreciate life's beauty as it unfolds.

Mindful listening is another technique that encourages presence and connection. You cultivate empathy and understanding by genuinely listening to others without interrupting or planning your response, enriching your relationships and spiritual life.

Integrating meditation and mindfulness into daily life can be seamless and rewarding. Consider practicing mindfulness during routine tasks, such as washing dishes or drinking tea. Pay attention to the sensations, smells, and sounds, allowing these activities to become meditative experiences.

Meditation apps can also benefit you by offering guided sessions that fit your schedule. These tools provide variety and structure, making it easier to maintain a regular practice. Whether a few minutes of mindfulness or a more extended meditation session, incorporating these practices into your routine can transform your day, bringing peace and spiritual insight.

Reflection Section: Starting Your Meditation Journey

Take a moment to consider how you might begin or deepen your meditation practice. Set aside a dedicated space in your home that invites calm and reflection. Choose a time each day to sit quietly and focus on your breath, using a meditation app if it helps guide you. Reflect on the difference these practices make in your life, noticing the peace and clarity they bring. As you explore meditation, let it become a gentle companion on your path to spiritual growth and inner peace.

FINDING MEANING AND PURPOSE IN AGING

As the years pass, many reflect on the more profound questions we might ask about life. This period of reflection often prompts a search for meaning and purpose, a spiritual exploration that can bring profound fulfillment. Aging naturally encourages this quest, as transitions such as retirement, changes in family roles, or shifts in health prompt a reevaluation of priorities.

It is a time to align actions with personal values, ensuring that what you do resonates with *who you are*. This alignment enhances inner peace and imbues daily life with a sense of direction and intention.

Discovering one's life purpose is personal, but some strategies can guide this exploration. Journaling is an effective tool, offering a space to uncover passions and interests that may have been over-looked. Simple prompts, like writing about activities that bring joy or examining past experiences that felt meaningful, can reveal patterns and insights.

Engaging in activities that reflect core beliefs can also illuminate your path. Whether volunteering for a cause you care about or participating in a hobby that ignites your spirit, these pursuits can affirm your purpose and provide clarity.

Service and contribution play a significant role in finding purpose, as giving back enriches both the giver and the receiver. Volunteering in community service projects offers a tangible way to make a difference, connecting you with others who share your commitment to common goals. Mentoring younger generations through formal programs or informal interactions allows you to share your wisdom and experiences, leaving a lasting impact. Such acts of service not only contribute to the well-being of others but also nourish your spirit, fostering a deep sense of fulfillment and human connection.

Many have found renewed purpose later in life, embarking on new ventures or initiatives that reflect their evolving interests and values. Take, for example, a retired teacher who began a literacy program for adults in her community, inspired by her lifelong passion for education. Her initiative provided valuable skills to participants and reignited her sense of purpose. Another individual, after a lengthy career in finance, turned to art, opening a gallery that highlights local talent. This new chapter brought joy and a sense of accomplishment as he discovered a way to blend his love for creativity with community engagement.

Personal accounts of spiritual transformation abound, illustrating how embracing purpose can lead to growth and self-discovery. Consider the story of a grandmother who found fulfillment in gardening after raising her family. Her backyard became a sanctuary for her peace of mind and neighbors who visited to share in the beauty and bounty of her garden. Her journey reflects the power of pursuing passions and how they can transform the individual *and* those around them.

These stories and experiences demonstrate that purpose is not confined to any age or stage of life. Purpose evolves with us, reflecting our changing interests, circumstances, and insights. By exploring what brings meaning to your life and aligning your actions with your values, you can find a sense of fulfillment that enriches your days and extends beyond yourself.

Through reflection, service, and the pursuit of passions, the quest for purpose becomes a rich range of experiences and connections, offering spiritual and personal growth.

SPIRITUAL PRACTICES ACROSS CULTURES

Imagine standing on the shores of the Ganges River in India, the air filled with the scent of incense and the sound of chanting. This is where yoga originated, a spiritual practice that has lasted centuries. Yoga is more than physical movement; it is a unifying practice that harmonizes the body, mind, and spirit. It encourages introspection, helping practitioners find peace and balance daily.

Across the globe, in China, Qigong offers another path to spiritual wellness. This practice combines movement, meditation, and controlled breathing to cultivate and balance life energy. It emphasizes the interconnectedness of all things, fostering a sense of peace and alignment with the universe.

Both yoga and Qigong offer profound insights into the power of integrating physical and spiritual practices.

Indigenous cultures worldwide also have rich spiritual traditions that connect deeply to the Earth and the cosmos. These rituals and ceremonies often celebrate life cycles and transitions, marking noteworthy events with reverence and gratitude.

For instance, Native American sweat lodges serve as purification rituals, promoting healing and spiritual renewal. Participants enter the lodge, a structure symbolizing the womb of the Earth, to pray and meditate, emerging with a renewed sense of clarity and purpose. Similarly, the Maori of New Zealand engage in the haka, a traditional dance that embodies their spiritual beliefs and connection to their ancestors.

These practices remind us of the timeless human desire to connect with something greater than ourselves.

Despite their diversity, spiritual practices across cultures share universal themes of connection, transcendence, and inner peace. Nature often plays a vital role in these practices, bridging the physical and spiritual worlds. Many traditions encourage spending time outdoors, where the natural world teaches patience, resilience, and harmony.

Whether it is a quiet walk through the forest or a moment of reflection by the ocean, nature invites us to slow down and listen to the wisdom around us. Rituals that mark life's transitions, such as births, marriages, and deaths, also highlight the cyclical nature of existence, reminding us of the continuity and interconnectedness of all life.

Incorporating elements from diverse spiritual practices into your life will enrich your spiritual journey. Start by exploring practices that resonate with you through books, documentaries, or cultural events. Creating a personalized spiritual routine allows you to blend elements from different traditions, tailoring them to your beliefs and lifestyle.

You might begin with yoga poses to start your day, followed by a Qigong session to center your energy. Participating in cultural workshops or retreats can also deepen your understanding and appreciation of these practices. These experiences offer opportunities to learn from skilled practitioners and immerse yourself in the cultural context of the practices you are exploring.

Many individuals have experienced profound spiritual growth through cultural immersion. Consider the story of a woman who traveled to Japan and participated in a Zen meditation retreat. The experience transformed her perspective, offering insights into mindfulness and simplicity that she carried into her daily life. Another individual spiritually awakened during a pilgrimage to the Camino de Santiago in Spain. She was walking the ancient path, which provided space for reflection and connection, fostering a sense of peace and purpose.

Such accounts illustrate the transformative power of spiritual practices around the planet, showing how they can deepen our understanding of ourselves and the world around us.

EMBRACING REFLECTION AND LIFE REVIEW

Reflecting on past experiences often leads to a deeper understanding of oneself, fostering spiritual insight and growth. When we take the time to look back, we revisit the paths we have traveled and gain a clearer picture of *who* we are and what we have learned.

Reflection allows us to join the dots of our lives, linking moments of joy and sorrow into a cohesive narrative that enriches our understanding of our place in the world. This process is not merely about reminiscing; it is an active engagement with our past that can reveal hidden strengths, teach valuable lessons, and guide us toward a more enlightened future.

Engaging in guided self-reflection techniques, such as asking specific questions about pivotal life events or considering the emotions tied to memories, can facilitate this process. These reflective practices serve as powerful tools for emotional healing, as they bring clarity and acceptance, helping us to let go of past burdens and embrace the present with a greater sense of peace.

Conducting a "life review" provides a structured way to examine significant life events and milestones. This process involves creating a life map or timeline, visually representing the key moments that have shaped your journey. Plotting these events allows you to see patterns emerge, providing insights into how experiences have influenced your development.

Reflective writing exercises further deepen this exploration by encouraging you to articulate the lessons learned from each milestone. Writing about how these experiences have influenced your values and beliefs will illuminate paths you wish to pursue or changes you want to make. Through this introspective journey, you gain a greater appreciation of your life's narrative and its wisdom.

Storytelling is a vital component of the life review process, offering a means to share your journey with others. By recording personal narratives, you preserve the stories of your life for your family or community, creating a legacy that lasts for generations. Engaging in oral history projects or legacy interviews can bring these stories to life, fostering connection and understanding. Sharing your experiences not only strengthens bonds with loved ones but also provides them with valuable insights into your character and values. These narratives serve as a bridge between the past and the future, offering guidance and inspiration to those who follow you.

Embracing the lessons learned through reflection is essential for shaping your spiritual path. By setting intentions based on past experiences, you can align your actions with the insights gained, inspiring growth and fulfillment. Reflecting on the challenges overcome and the strengths developed along the way empowers you to apply these lessons to current and future endeavors.

This continuous learning and adaptation process enriches your spiritual journey and enhances your resilience and adaptability to life's inevitable changes. As you integrate these insights into your daily life, you cultivate a more profound sense of purpose and peace, guiding you toward a more meaningful and connected existence.

In conclusion, the reflection and life review process is a powerful personal and spiritual growth tool. By thinking about the experiences that have shaped us and sharing our stories with others, we gain insight and understanding, making deeper connections and giving us a more profound sense of purpose.

8

NAVIGATING HEALTH CHALLENGES

I recall meeting a vibrant woman named Eleanor at a community event who had just turned seventy. Despite enduring chronic back pain for years, she caught my attention with her lively spirit and zest for life. Eleanor's secret was her comprehensive approach to pain management. She shared how she had embraced alternative therapies instead of solely relying on medications, which often came with unwanted side effects. Her story highlights the power of treating the body, focusing on symptoms and overall well-being.

Chronic pain affects millions of people globally, and traditional treatments often involve medication, which can frequently lead to side effects that outweigh the benefits. Holistic approaches offer promising alternatives.

Acupuncture, for instance, is an ancient practice that involves inserting thin needles into specific points on the body to balance energy flow or stimulate nerves and muscles for pain relief. Many find it effective in reducing pain and improving circulation without the adverse effects of drugs.

Similarly, chiropractic adjustments focus on aligning the musculoskeletal system, particularly the spine, to relieve pain and enhance function. These adjustments can help alleviate discomfort by addressing the root causes of pain rather than just masking it.

Mind-body techniques also gain recognition for managing pain by reducing stress and tension. As we have seen, meditation is a simple yet powerful practice that encourages relaxation and mindfulness, helping to ease muscle tension and lower stress levels. This, in turn, can lead to a decrease in pain perception. Guided imagery, which involves visualizing calming and peaceful images, can also be an effective tool for pain reduction. This technique uses the power of the mind to influence physical sensations, creating a sense of control over pain.

Biofeedback sessions provide another avenue for managing pain. By learning to regulate physiological responses such as heart rate and muscle tension, individuals can gain greater control over their body's reactions to pain.

Lifestyle changes play a crucial role in supporting pain management. An anti-inflammatory diet, rich in fruits, vegetables, whole grains, and omega-3 fatty acids, can help reduce inflammation, a common contributor to chronic pain. Foods like leafy greens, berries, and fatty fish are excellent choices.

Regular low-impact exercise like swimming or walking can help maintain mobility and reduce stiffness. These activities are gentle on the joints and promote circulation, alleviating pain and improving overall health. Incorporating these habits into your daily routine can significantly improve pain management and quality of life.

A personalized pain management plan tailored to your needs and circumstances makes all the difference. Collaborating with healthcare professionals, such as pain specialists or holistic practitioners, can help you develop your best strategy. They can guide you in integrating various therapies and lifestyle changes into your routine. A pain diary is a valuable tool for tracking triggers and effective treatments. By noting when pain occurs and what alleviates it, you can gain insights into patterns and make informed decisions about your management plan.

Reflection Section: Creating Your Personalized Pain Management Plan

Consider starting a pain diary to track your symptoms, triggers, and the effectiveness of different treatments. Write down observations each day, noting what activities or therapies bring relief. Reflect on whether holistic methods like acupuncture or meditation might benefit you. Discuss these options with your healthcare provider to tailor a plan that fits your lifestyle and needs.

Taking this proactive approach means you will take control of your pain management journey, enhancing your well-being and quality of life.

NATURAL REMEDIES FOR COMMON AILMENTS

How about a comforting cup of ginger tea, its steam gently rising as you take in its spicy-sweet aroma? Known for its ability to ease nausea and soothe digestive discomfort, ginger has been cherished for centuries in many cultures. Its anti-inflammatory properties make it a natural choice for those seeking relief from common ailments without relying solely on conventional medications.

Similarly, lavender oil offers a soothing balm for the soul. A few drops on your pillow can promote relaxation and encourage restful sleep, helping you unwind after a long day. These natural remedies are not just folk tales but are backed by sound evidence and time-tested traditions that offer gentle yet effective relief.

Herbal supplements also play a significant role in managing health, particularly as we age. With its vibrant golden hue, turmeric is more than just a spice; it is a potent anti-inflammatory agent. The active ingredient, curcumin, has been studied for its ability to reduce inflammation, offering potential benefits for conditions like arthritis.

Similarly, echinacea is believed to boost the immune system. Often used at the onset of a cold, it can help reduce the duration and severity of symptoms, offering a natural defense against seasonal illnesses.

These herbs provide a supportive role in health management, allowing for a more integrated approach to wellness.

When considering natural remedies, consulting healthcare providers before starting new treatments is crucial. "Natural" does not always mean *safe*—especially when mixed with prescription medications. Some herbs can interact with drugs, altering their effectiveness or causing unexpected side effects. For example, taking the herbal remedy St John's wort for symptoms of depression can make you photosensitive.

It is essential to discuss any supplements you are considering with your doctor to ensure they fit within your overall health plan. Understanding appropriate dosages and administration methods is also necessary. Herbs can be potent, and taking too much can lead to adverse effects. Following guidelines and seeking professional advice will help to ensure these remedies complement your health regimen *safely*.

Natural treatments are deeply ingrained in many cultural and historical practices. Traditional Chinese medicine, for instance, has long utilized herbs and acupuncture to promote balance and health. This comprehensive approach considers the body an interconnected system, treating ailments by restoring harmony rather than just addressing symptoms.

Indigenous cultures around the world have relied on plant-based healing methods for generations. These practices passed down through stories and rituals, highlight a profound respect for nature's healing ability. From the Amazon's range of medicinal plants, including cannabis, to the North American sage used in cleansing ceremonies, such traditions offer valuable insights into the potential of natural remedies.

Reflection Section: Exploring Natural Remedies

Consider exploring natural remedies that resonate with you. Start by researching options like ginger tea or lavender oil and discuss them with your healthcare provider. Keep a journal to note any changes or improvements you observe. This mindful approach allows you to integrate natural remedies into your wellness routine thoughtfully *and* safely.

BUILDING A SUPPORTIVE HEALTHCARE TEAM

Your healthcare team is like an orchestra, and each player is essential in creating their part in a harmonious symphony to support your well-being. Just as the conductor ensures every instrument plays its part, a primary care physician can guide your healthcare journey, coordinating with specialists to provide a seamless experience.

This collaborative approach means working with various professionals, like nutritionists who can tailor dietary advice to your needs or physical therapists who design exercise regimens to keep you moving without pain. Having a team ensures that all aspects of your health are considered—not just the immediate issues. This comprehensive care is vital for addressing the complexities of aging, allowing you to continue to thrive.

Choosing the right healthcare providers requires thoughtful consideration. It is essential to look beyond the surface and evaluate their credentials and areas of expertise. You want professionals who understand the unique challenges of aging. Communication style matters as well. You deserve someone who listens and takes time to answer your questions, making you feel heard and respected. Patient reviews can offer insight into a provider's reputation and how they relate to those in their care. A good fit will align with your personal health goals and values, with the chance to develop a trusting relationship where your concerns are respected and taken seriously.

Clear communication with your healthcare team is crucial for adequate care. Before appointments, prepare a list of questions and concerns. This ensures that you cover all the topics important to you, making the most of your time with your provider. Keeping thorough records of treatments and outcomes helps track your progress and informs future decisions. These records are a valuable resource, providing a clear picture of your health history. Bringing these details to appointments can facilitate more informed discussions with your healthcare team, ensuring everyone is on the same page and working towards the same goals.

Being proactive in making your healthcare choices empowers you to take control of your health. Researching treatment options and alternatives allows you to make informed decisions rather than relying solely on recommendations. This knowledge is power, giving you confidence in the path you choose. Do not hesitate to seek second opinions when necessary. Another perspective can offer new insights or confirm your current plan, providing peace of mind.

Taking an active role in healthcare means advocating for yourself and ensuring your needs and preferences guide your decisions.

Case Study: Navigating a Collaborative Healthcare Approach

Consider Martha, who found herself facing a complex medical issue. She assembled a healthcare team that included her primary care doctor, a nutritionist, and a physical therapist. Each played a role in her care, from dietary adjustments to tailored exercise plans. Communication with her and her team was *vital*. Martha kept a detailed health journal, which she shared with her team, ensuring everyone was aligned on her progress and treatment. Her proactive approach and willingness to seek the best care transformed her health journey, leading to improved outcomes and greater control over her well-being.

SIMPLIFYING MEDICATION MANAGEMENT

Managing multiple medications can feel overwhelming, especially when prescriptions change or are added over time. Many of you might have experienced the frustration of missing a dose or even forgetting whether you took a medication. To make this easier, consider using pill organizers.

These simple tools can help you keep track of daily doses and ensure no medication is missed. Pill organizers come in assorted designs, ranging from basic weekly layouts to more complex ones that accommodate multiple doses per day. They benefit those with memory concerns, offering a straightforward way to manage medication schedules without stress.

In our 21st century digital age, technology is an excellent ally in medication management. Smartphone apps and alarms are reliable reminders to take medications immediately. Many apps are designed for medication management, allowing you to input your prescriptions and schedules and set alerts. This approach helps you remember doses and records your medication history, which can be shared with healthcare providers.

Alarms, whether on your phone or a dedicated device, act as gentle nudges, ensuring that medication is taken consistently, thus maintaining the effectiveness of your treatment plan.

Understanding medication instructions is crucial to ensure you receive your prescriptions' full benefit without unintended side effects. It is essential to clarify any doubts with your pharmacist, who can explain how each medication should be taken. They can inform you about interactions with other drugs or foods, which is vital for avoiding adverse effects.

Reviewing potential side effects is also essential. Knowing what to expect, you can monitor your body's responses and contact a healthcare provider if something feels off. This understanding empowers you to take medications safely and effectively, fostering a proactive approach to your health.

Regular medication reviews are beneficial for optimizing your treatment regimen. Periodic assessments with your healthcare provider can help determine if each medication is necessary and practical. During these reviews, you can discuss any side effects or changes in your condition. This dialogue can lead to prescription adjustments that better suit your health needs. Evaluating the effectiveness of medications ensures that you are not taking unnecessary drugs, which can reduce the risk of interactions and side effects. It also allows exploring alternative treatments if a medication does not deliver the desired results.

Keeping organized records of your medications is a practical way to manage your health. Creating a medication chart or list that includes each drug's name, dose, and timing will provide a quick reference. This list should be updated regularly, especially after any changes in prescriptions.

Sharing this information with caregivers or family members can also be helpful, ensuring that everyone involved in your care is informed. Accurate documentation is valuable during medical appointments, allowing healthcare providers to make informed decisions about your treatment.

As we conclude this chapter, remember that medication management is integral to maintaining health. Adopting these strategies ensures that your medications serve you well, contributing to a healthier, more balanced life.

9

TECHNOLOGY AND AGING

One evening, while sipping tea, my granddaughter showed me how to use an "app" to share photos instantly. Her fingers flew over my "tablet" screen, leaving me both amazed and slightly bewildered. That moment was a revelation. It reminded me of the incredible power of technology to bring us closer—no matter the miles between us. Innovative technology can often seem daunting, but it is *critical* to staying connected and engaged in our rapidly evolving world.

In our digital age, mastering basic digital skills can open doors to new experiences and relationships, enriching your life in various unexpected ways.

Digital literacy is a gateway to maintaining social connections and accessing vital information. Imagine being able to send an email to a friend across the country, sharing updates and pictures with a few clicks. Or consider using social media to connect with family and friends, catch up on their lives, and share your own stories.

Platforms like Facebook and Instagram allow you to see photos, comment on posts, and exchange messages easily. These tools transform how we connect, making it more immediate and personal. The ability to communicate through video calls adds another layer, enabling you to see the faces and hear the voices of loved ones, making every conversation more intimate and meaningful! Video calling platforms such as Zoom or Facetime have become integral to our lives, especially when physical visits are challenging. They bridge the gap, ensuring you remain active in your family's life if they are distant.

Mastering a few essential skills is vital to act within this digital landscape. Let us look at a few technical matters you can master quickly and join in the communication!

Setting up and using an email account is a fundamental step. It allows you to send and receive messages, stay informed about events, and manage subscriptions. Start by choosing a reliable email provider like Gmail or Yahoo. Follow the instructions to create your account, setting a strong, memorable password for security. Once set up, practice sending a simple email to a friend or family member.

Social media platforms, while vast, are manageable with some guidance. Begin by creating a profile on Facebook or Instagram, entering basic information, and uploading a photo if you wish. Explore the platform by searching for friends or groups that align with your interests. Each platform has a Help section and tutorials to guide you.

Improving digital literacy may seem tricky, but resources abound to support your journey. Many local libraries and community centers offer tech workshops specifically designed for seniors. These sessions cover everything from basic computer skills to navigating the internet safely. They provide hands-on experience in a supportive environment, allowing you to learn independently.

Online platforms like Coursera and Udemy offer tutorials and courses on various digital skills, from setting up social media accounts to mastering video calls. These resources are accessible from the comfort of your home, offering flexibility in learning. The National Council on Aging, in partnership with AT&T, has also launched a digital literacy initiative, offering self-paced modules and in-person workshops to enhance your skills.

In our fast-paced tech world, ongoing learning and adapting are fundamental skills. Staying current with evolving technologies ensures you remain connected and informed. Subscribing to tech newsletters will provide regular updates on new tools and trends, keeping you in the loop. These newsletters often offer tips and advice tailored for seniors, making technology much more approachable for us!

Joining online forums or groups focused on technology for seniors can also be beneficial. These communities provide a platform to ask questions, share experiences, and learn from others on a similar learning curve. Engaging with these resources enhances your skills and builds confidence, empowering you to embrace technology as a tool for connection and enrichment.

Interactive Element: Technology Comfort Checklist

Reflect on your current comfort level with digital technology. Consider the following checklist to guide your exploration:

- **Email Setup**: Have you created an email account? Are you comfortable sending and receiving emails?

- **Social Media Navigation**: Have you created a profile on a platform like Facebook? Do you know how to search for friends and groups?
- **Video-Calling**: Have you tried using a video-calling platform like Zoom or Facetime? Are you comfortable initiating and ending calls?
- **Learning Resources**: Have you explored any local tech workshops or online courses? Are there specific skills you would like to learn more about?

Use this checklist to identify areas where you feel confident and where you might seek further guidance or practice.

ESSENTIAL TECHNOLOGY TOOLS FOR EVERYDAY LIFE

Picture this scene: waking up in the morning, and with a simple voice command, your favorite music starts playing, the lights gently brighten, and your coffee machine begins brewing! This is the magic of smart home devices, such as voice-activated assistants like Amazon's Alexa or Google Home.

These devices can simplify daily tasks, making life more convenient and enjoyable. They can help you easily manage your schedule, set reminders, and even control home appliances. Imagine saying, "Alexa, remind me to take my medication at 2 pm," and having your assistant ensure you *never* miss an important task. These tools are designed to integrate seamlessly into your life, helping at the very sound of your voice.

Technology's role in health and wellness is equally transformative. Wearable fitness trackers, like Fitbit or Apple Watch, have become famous for monitoring physical activity levels. They track steps, heart rate, and even sleep patterns, providing insights into your daily health habits. These devices motivate you to stay active by setting goals and celebrating achievements.

For mental well-being, apps like Calm or Headspace offer guided meditation and relaxation exercises. These apps are like having your mindfulness coach, helping you manage stress and find moments of peace amid the hustle and bustle of life.

Integrating these technologies allows you to take proactive steps toward a healthier physical and mental lifestyle.

Technology again opens a world of new possibilities regarding entertainment and leisure. Streaming services like Netflix or Spotify provide endless options for movies, TV shows, and music, all accessible at the touch of a button. Whether watching a classic film, a new blockbuster, or discovering contemporary music, these platforms cater to diverse tastes, ensuring there is always "something for everyone"!

For those who love reading, e-readers like Kindle or audiobook platforms like Audible offer a library in your pocket. You can enjoy your favorite books anytime, anywhere, without needing physical storage. These tools will enrich your leisure time, making it easy to indulge in hobbies and entertainment *whenever* you like.

Choosing the right technology tools involves understanding your needs and preferences. When evaluating products, consider features that align with your lifestyle. For instance, if you enjoy listening to music while cooking, a smart speaker with good sound quality might be ideal. Reading reviews from other users can provide valuable insights into a product's performance and reliability.

Once you select a device, setting it up and customizing it to your liking is vital. Take the time to explore its features, adjust settings, and personalize it to suit your routines. Many devices come with user-friendly guides or customer support to assist you through the process, ensuring a smooth and hassle-free experience.

Interactive Element: Technology Selection Checklist

Reflect on the technology tools that will enhance your daily life. Consider the following questions to guide your choices:

- **Convenience**: Do you need assistance managing daily tasks, such as setting reminders or controlling home devices?
- **Health and Wellness**: Are you interested in tracking fitness activities or exploring meditation and stress management apps?
- **Entertainment**: What are your preferences for streaming services or reading platforms?

Use these questions to identify the tools that best align with your lifestyle. Explore reviews and user experiences to make informed decisions.

BRIDGING THE TECH GAP: LEARNING AT ANY AGE

Many older adults face unique challenges when it comes to adopting the use of modern technology. You are expected to feel intimidated and hesitate, especially if digital tools have not been part of your daily life for many years. You might worry about making mistakes or even accidentally damaging a device. This fear can create a barrier, making it challenging to embrace technology's benefits. Resistance to change is natural for humans, but it is essential to remember that technology will improve and enhance your life in many ways. By approaching it with an open mind, you can overcome these challenges and discover new ways to connect, learn, and enjoy life!

One effective strategy for mastering modern technology is to break down complex tasks into smaller, manageable steps. When faced with a new device or program, take it one step at a time. **Start with the basics, like turning the device on and off, and gradu-**ally move on to more complex functions. Practicing regularly is vital to building confidence and competence. Set aside a little time each day to explore and familiarize yourself with the technology, allowing yourself to learn at your own pace. Steady practice helps reinforce your skills, making the process less overwhelming and *rewarding*. Technology is designed to be used intuitively, and with patience, you will find that you can navigate it with ease!

Intergenerational learning is a powerful way to enhance your tech skills. Collaborating with younger family members or friends provides invaluable support and encouragement. Grandchildren **often have a natural aptitude for technology and can offer guid-**ance in a way that is both patient and fun! Consider setting up regular tech sessions where they can teach you about new apps, devices, or features. Engaging in family tech projects or challenges, **such as creating a digital photo album or exploring virtual muse-**ums, can be a delightful way to play and learn together.

Interactions like this not only enhance your tech skills but also strengthen family bonds, creating shared experiences that are both educational *and* enjoyable.

You can bridge the tech gap and enjoy technology's many benefits. Whether it is connecting with loved ones, exploring new hobbies, or simply making daily tasks easier, technology has the potential to enrich your life in countless ways.

The key is approaching it with curiosity and patience, knowing that learning is lifelong. Each new skill you acquire opens fresh possibilities, inviting you to explore the digital world with increasing confidence and positive enthusiasm.

ONLINE SAFETY AND PRIVACY: PROTECTING YOUR INFORMATION

As we engage more with technology, the privacy and safety risks of digital interactions increase. Identity theft, for example, is a growing concern, where malicious actors can steal your data, leading to unauthorized access to your accounts and even economic loss. Phishing attempts, another prevalent threat, often come in the form of deceptive emails or messages designed to trick you into revealing sensitive information such as passwords or credit card numbers. Being vigilant and discerning about the communications you receive can protect you from these frauds.

Recognizing these threats is the first step toward a safer online experience.

Enhancing your online security begins with creating strong, unique passwords *for each* online account. A good password combines letters, numbers, and symbols and should not be easily guessable. Avoid using simple words or sequences, like "password123" or "abcd1234" or your birth date.

Consider using a password manager to keep track of your passwords securely. This tool generates and stores passwords, ensuring they remain unique and complex. Enabling two-factor authentication (2FA) adds an extra layer of protection. With 2FA, accessing your accounts requires a password and a second verification form, such as a code sent to your phone. This makes it significantly harder for unauthorized users to gain access, even if they have your password.

To further protect yourself, adopting secure internet behaviors is essential. Begin by identifying secure websites. Before entering personal information, look for "https" at the beginning of the URL and a padlock icon in the address bar. These indicators mean the website encrypts your data, making it more secure. Be wary of websites that lack these features.

Additionally, regularly review the privacy settings on your social media platforms. These settings control who can see your posts and personal information. Adjust them to limit access to only people you trust, reducing the risk of misusing or sharing your data without consent. Staying informed about your privacy settings helps maintain control over your online presence.

Staying informed about online safety is also an ongoing process. Subscribing to cybersecurity blogs or newsletters will provide valuable insights into the latest threats and how to counteract them. These resources offer practical advice and updates on new security measures, helping you avoid potential risks. Participating in online safety webinars or workshops can also enhance your understanding of cybersecurity. These sessions are designed to teach you about common threats and prevention techniques, offering guidance tailored to various levels of technological proficiency. Organizations like ConnectSafely provide comprehensive guides and resources to help you navigate the digital world securely.

Online safety and privacy are integral to your enjoyable, peaceful digital life. Adopting these practices will protect your personal information and gain confidence in navigating the digital world. Your journey through technology is unique; with these tools, you can embrace it with security and peace of mind.

10

CULTURAL PERSPECTIVES ON AGING

As I shared a coffee with a friend who had just returned from a journey to Sardinia, Italy, she shared stories of vibrant centenarians, their laughter echoing through the cobblestone streets. These elders, she noted, embodied vitality and community spirit, living testaments to a life of well-being. Her tales reminded me of "Blue Zones," regions scattered across the globe where people live longer and *thrive* well into their golden years. These areas reveal secrets of longevity that transcend genetics, rooted instead in lifestyle and cultural practices that foster health and happiness. They offer lessons that, when embraced, can enrich our lives, no matter where we reside.

LESSONS FROM THE BLUE ZONES: LONGEVITY SECRETS

The term "Blue Zones" was coined from a National Geographic expedition led by Dan Buettner, seeking to uncover the mysteries behind the world's longest-lived populations. Among these regions, Okinawa in Japan stands out for its keen sense of community and purpose, known locally as "Ikigai," which translates to "reason for being." Here, elders maintain close ties with family and neighbors, often meeting to share meals and stories. This sense of belonging and purpose contributes to their exceptional lifespan, as does their plant-based diet rich in tofu, sweet potatoes, and turmeric.

Similarly, Ikaria in Greece offers insights into its Mediterranean diet, emphasizing fresh vegetables, olive oil, and moderate wine consumption. This island, where naps are part of the daily routine, has become synonymous with heart health and longevity.

In Sardinia, Italy, the secret lies in strong family ties and an active lifestyle. The Sardinians engage in regular physical activities, often as part of their daily work or leisure, such as shepherding or gardening. Their diet, which includes whole grains, legumes, and lean meats, complements this active way of life.

These Blue Zones share common threads—plant-based diets, regular movement, and robust social networks—that paint a picture of a life balanced between body, mind, and community. These factors collectively contribute to not only a *longer* life—but a more *fulfilling* one.

These Blue Zones' social and cultural elements offer profound insights into aging with grace and dignity. In Okinawa, "moai," or social support groups, are crucial in providing emotional *and* financial backing. These groups offer companionship and a safety net during life's inevitable challenges. In Ikaria, the slower pace of life and a solid cultural attitude that respects elders create an environment where aging is a celebrated journey rather than any decline. Sardinians also profoundly appreciate their elders, who remain integral to family and community life, ensuring that wisdom is handed down through generations.

Incorporating these principles into your life can foster better health and a more profound sense of fulfillment. Start by reflecting on your personal "Ikigai."

What activities or relationships bring you joy and purpose each day?

Cultivate these elements through hobbies, volunteering, or spending time with loved ones. Building and nurturing social networks is equally vital. Engage in community activities, join clubs, or contact friends and family regularly. These connections enrich your life with support and companionship.

Reflection Section: Embracing Blue Zone Habits

Take a moment to consider how you can integrate Blue Zone habits into your routine. Reflect on your current lifestyle and identify areas for potential change. Could you incorporate more plant-based meals into your diet? Is there a local group or activity that interests you? Write down a few steps you can take this week to embrace these longevity secrets. Perhaps plan a meal inspired by the Mediterranean diet or arrange a walk with a friend. These minor adjustments lead to a healthier, more connected life.

TRADITIONAL PRACTICES FOR MODERN AGING

In the heart of India, the ancient science of Ayurveda has thrived for centuries, offering an integrated approach to health that focuses on balance and harmony within the body. This tradition emphasizes the importance of diet, lifestyle, and mental well-being in maintaining health and longevity. Ayurvedic practices revolve around the concept of "Doshas," which are biological energies believed to govern physiological activity. By understanding one's unique constitution, or "Prakruti," individuals can tailor their diet and lifestyle to support optimal health. For instance, incorporating spices like turmeric and ginger into meals can enhance digestion and bolster immunity, reflecting Ayurveda's focus on conscious eating and balance.

Similarly, Traditional Chinese Medicine (TCM) offers another time-honored approach to health, rooted in the concept of "Qi," or life energy, which flows through the body. TCM practitioners believe that illness arises when this energy flow is disrupted. Techniques such as acupuncture and herbal remedies restore balance and promote well-being. Acupuncture, with its precise needle placement, stimulates specific points in the body to enhance energy flow and alleviate pain. This practice, often combined with modern pain management techniques, provides a comprehensive approach to treating arthritis and migraines. Herbal medicine, another cornerstone of TCM, complements conventional treatments by offering natural alternatives for managing chronic conditions.

Rituals play a vital role in maintaining health and well-being across cultures.

In Japan, the tea ceremony is not just about drinking tea; it is a meditative practice that fosters mindfulness and tranquility. The careful preparation and consumption of tea has become a form of meditation, encouraging participants to be present in the moment and reflect on the beauty of simplicity. This ritual, deeply embedded in Japanese culture, offers a respite from the hustle of daily life, promoting mental clarity and relaxation.

In Africa, dance rituals serve as a form of physical fitness and community bonding. Rhythmic movements and communal participation strengthen social ties and enhance physical health, highlighting the dual benefits of such practices.

Cultural significance imbues these traditions with profound meaning.

Native American healing rituals, for example, are deeply spiritual, linking physical health to the community's and the environment's well-being. These practices often involve ceremonies that honor the interconnectedness of all living things, reinforcing a sense of belonging and purpose.

Similarly, in Nordic countries, sauna bathing is more than a method of relaxation; it is a communal activity that fosters social interaction and strengthens family bonds. The warmth of the sauna, coupled with the tradition of social gathering, creates an environment conducive to open communication and shared experiences.

These ancient practices offer invaluable insights into how cultural traditions can support modern aging. By integrating these time-honored methods with contemporary health practices, you can create a personalized approach to well-being that resonates with your lifestyle. Consider incorporating elements of Ayurveda or TCM into your daily routine, such as herbal teas or mindful eating habits. Engage in a simple ritual, like a daily walk or meditation, to center your thoughts and rejuvenate your spirit.

These small but meaningful practices can enhance your physical *and* mental health, weaving wisdom from the past into the fabric of your everyday life.

Reflection Section: Integrating Tradition

Reflect on which traditional practices resonate with you. Is there a ritual or cultural practice you would like to explore further? Consider dedicating a few moments each day to a new practice, whether a calming tea ritual or a gentle series of yoga stretches.

Note any changes in your well-being as you incorporate these elements into your life.

GLOBAL WISDOM: AGING GRACEFULLY ACROSS CULTURES

In the heart of many Indigenous cultures, elders hold a revered status that transcends their years. They are seen as the keepers of wisdom, the storytellers who pass down the rich tapestry of their history to younger generations.

This reverence for elders is not just about age but about the wealth of experience and knowledge they embody. In many Native American communities, elders are critical in guiding youth through life's complexities, using storytelling to impart lessons and values. These stories are more than mere tales; they are the building blocks of cultural identity, shaping the community's moral and ethical framework.

This storytelling tradition, a cornerstone in Aboriginal cultures, also bridges the past and present, ensuring that the "wisdom of the ancients" remains alive—and relevant.

In African tribes, elders are often seen as community leaders, not merely because of their age but due to their accumulated wisdom and experience. They are the custodians of cultural heritage; their counsel is sought during decision-making and conflict resolution. This respect for older adults is a testament to the deep-rooted belief in the interconnectedness of all stages of life. It reflects the African philosophy of "ubuntu," which emphasizes community, shared humanity, and the idea that one's well-being is intrinsically linked to the well-being of others.

Elders in these communities are not just leaders; they embody resilience and adaptability, guiding their communities through the changing tides of modern life.

Across the globe, cultural values profoundly shape the experience of aging. In many Eastern cultures, aging is embraced as a natural and honorable phase of life, when individuals are celebrated for their accumulated wisdom and contributions. In contrast, Western societies often idolize youth, sometimes neglecting the value and beauty that comes with age.

This dichotomy can influence how individuals perceive their aging process. In Eastern cultures, older individuals often remain active participants in family and community life, and their opinions and experiences are deeply valued. This cultural attitude fosters a sense of purpose and belonging, contributing to mental and emotional health.

Incorporating these global perspectives into your life can enhance *your* aging experience, offering richness and depth. Practicing gratitude and humility, as seen in Buddhist teachings, can help cultivate a sense of peace and acceptance. These practices encourage you to appreciate the present while acknowledging the wisdom gained from past experiences.

Engaging in community service is another way to stay connected and give back. You can share your skills and knowledge by volunteering or participating in local initiatives, forging new connections, and strengthening community bonds.

Reflection Section: Embracing Global Wisdom

Reflect on how you view aging and the influence of your cultural background. Consider what aspects of these diverse cultural attitudes resonate with you. Could you incorporate new traditions or practices to enrich your experience? You could start a small story-telling circle with family, sharing stories from your past that impart lessons or values. Or try volunteering on a local community project where your insights would be invaluable. Write down a few ideas that inspire you, and take a moment to appreciate the global wealth of wisdom surrounding us all.

ADAPTING CULTURAL PRACTICES FOR PERSONAL GROWTH

Cultural practices from around the world offer abundant knowledge and inspiration that can be adapted to improve our daily lives. By personalizing these practices, you can integrate their benefits into your routine, building a lifestyle that promotes well-being and personal growth.

Take, for instance, the Mediterranean diet, renowned for its heart health benefits. This diet emphasizes fresh vegetables, whole grains, and healthy fats like olive oil. Incorporating these elements into your meals allows you to enjoy delicious food while supporting cardiovascular health. The Mediterranean approach to dining—savoring meals with family and friends—also encourages slower eating and a greater appreciation of the food we consume.

Another example is the Japanese practice of "Ikebana," the art of flower arranging, which serves as a meditative and creative outlet. By engaging in Ikebana, you can cultivate mindfulness and develop a deeper connection with nature. The process of arranging flowers allows you to focus on balance, harmony, and simplicity, offering a peaceful respite from the busyness of life. It encourages you to find beauty in imperfection and embrace the transient nature of existence. This mindful activity will bring a sense of calm and creativity to your day, enriching your mental and emotional well-being.

Blending multiple cultural practices can lead to unique routines catering to your needs and preferences. Imagine creating a fusion exercise routine that combines the fluid movements of Tai Chi with the rhythmic strides of Nordic walking. Such a routine can offer the benefits of improved balance and cardiovascular health while providing a refreshing change of pace.

Similarly, you might design a daily routine incorporating yoga's flexibility and the Swedish "lagom" concept, emphasizing balance and moderation in all aspects of life. This combination promotes physical health while encouraging a balanced lifestyle, allowing you to enjoy life's pleasures without excess.

When adapting cultural practices into your life, it is essential to do so respectfully and thoughtfully. Understanding these practices' historical and cultural context can deepen your appreciation and ensure you honor their origins. Engaging with cultural communities or seeking authentic insights from practitioners will provide valuable guidance and enrich your experience. By approaching these practices with respect and openness, you also contribute to preserving and appreciating diverse cultural heritages.

Consider the story of an individual who embraced mindfulness through Zen Buddhism. Initially drawn to the philosophy and practice for its stress-reducing benefits, they found a more profound sense of peace and purpose by incorporating Zen principles into daily life. This personal journey of adaptation highlights how cultural practices can be tailored to fit individual lifestyles, leading to profound personal growth and fulfillment.

Communities adopting environmentally sustainable practices inspired by Indigenous wisdom also demonstrate successful cultural adaptation. By integrating traditional ecological knowledge with modern sustainability efforts, these communities have created harmonious environments that benefit both people *and* Earth.

As you explore these cultural practices, reflect on how they resonate with your values and goals. The richness of cultural diversity offers endless possibilities for personal growth and improved well-being. Welcome the opportunity to gain experience from these traditions, adapting them in ways that add to your life while respecting their origins. Doing so can create a lifestyle that nurtures your body, mind, and spirit.

11

INSPIRING STORIES AND PERSONAL GROWTH

One quiet morning recently, I was sharing brunch with an old friend, Susan, who had recently embarked on a remarkable new path. A retired schoolteacher, Susan, had always loved stories, but it was not until her late sixties that she decided to write one of her own. With a twinkle in her eye, over coffee, she shared how she had become a successful novelist, her books now adored by readers across the country! Susan's trek from classroom to bestseller list was challenging, but her passion for storytelling and determination to embrace change proved transformative. Her story shows that pursuing new dreams and desires is never too late.

In the same vein, consider the story of Jack, a former corporate executive who, after years in a high-pressure industry, traded his business suit for overalls to start an organic farm. Jack had always harbored a deep love for the land, a passion inherited from his grandfather. After retiring, Jack faced a crossroads: to continue consulting in his field or dive into something entirely new. Choosing the latter, he poured his energy into sustainable farming.

Today, his farm supplies local markets with fresh produce and serves as a community hub for teaching others about organic agriculture. Jack's shift "from the boardroom to barn" demonstrates how heartily welcoming new experiences can lead to profound personal fulfillment and broader impact.

Then there's Mary, a grandmother who returned to school to pursue a degree in art history. For years, she had painted as a hobby, often losing herself in the colors and textures of her canvases. When her family encouraged her to study art formally, Mary hesitated, unsure if she could meet the high demands of academic life. Yet, her love for art propelled her forward. Enrolling in a local university, Mary immersed herself in the history of artists who had inspired her work. After graduating with first-class honors, she now lectures at community centers, sharing her insights and encouraging others to appreciate the beauty and stories behind art. Mary's journey highlights the power of education and lifelong learning, showing how our passions can enrich our lives at any age.

Like many others, these individuals have thrived by being open to new experiences and challenges. They have embraced change, often jumping significant hurdles along the way. For some, this meant facing health issues head-on to achieve their goals. Susan, for instance, battled arthritis, which sometimes made typing painful. Yet, she adapted using voice-to-text software, ensuring her stories continued flowing. Jack faced financial constraints, using his savings to invest in the farm. His perseverance paid off as he slowly built a profitable enterprise. Mary juggled family responsibilities and coursework, finding balance through sheer determination *and* the support of her family.

Resilience and determination played crucial roles in all their journeys. Susan's persistence allowed her to overcome financial struggles, turning her writing into a successful career. Jack's story of starting anew in a different field exemplifies the courage to venture into the unknown. These real-life stories are about achieving "success" and the personal growth experienced. They encourage us to reflect on our strong potential for transformation, consider how we can accept change, and pursue our development.

Take a moment to think about your *own* life. What passions have you yet to explore further? What changes could lead to new and exciting paths? Consider journaling as a tool for reflection. Write about areas of personal interest and set achievable goals for growth. You are drawn to photography, teaching, or volunteering. Whatever it may be, remember that it is *never* too late to begin. Like Susan, Jack, and Mary, your journey is uniquely *yours* to shape and explore.

CELEBRATING MILESTONES: LESSONS FROM THE JOURNEY

Life is like a Persian carpet, woven with milestones, each one a symbol of the path we have followed. Celebrating these milestones honors our achievements and enhances our self-worth and satisfaction.

Imagine the warmth of gathering family and friends to commemorate a milestone birthday, the room filled with laughter and stories that span decades. Such celebrations are not just parties; they are affirmations of a life well-lived, reminders that every wrinkle and gray hair has a story to tell. Documenting these moments in a personal scrapbook or journal can be a cherished pastime, capturing the events, emotions, and *lessons* accompanying them. Flipping through these pages on a quiet afternoon can bring a sense of gratitude and pride, showing the resilience and determination that have carried you through life's many difficulties.

Take, for instance, the story of Ellen and Tom, a couple who celebrated their 50th wedding anniversary with a renewal of vows. Surrounded by loved ones, they reaffirmed their love and commitment, reflecting on the life they have built and are building together. Their celebration was a tribute to their enduring partnership and a reminder of the power of love and perseverance.

Similarly, there's David, who, at 70, fulfilled his lifelong dream of running a marathon. Crossing that finish line, he felt great accomplishment following years of training and dedication. These milestones are more than personal achievements; they are shared victories, inspiring those around us to pursue their dreams, regardless of age.

Reflecting on milestones can lead to valuable insights and life lessons. Patience and perseverance often emerge as common themes, illustrating the importance of *staying the course* even when the path is uncertain. Ellen and Tom's story highlights how a strong partnership can weather the storms of life, teaching us the value of intimate relationships and the strength found in the community. David's marathon tale underscores the power of setting long-term goals and the fulfillment that comes from achieving them. These reflections remind us that while the destination is necessary, the journey and lessons learned along the way truly enrich our lives.

Consider your milestones.

What achievements have marked your path? Whether it is a career milestone, a personal victory, or a moment of self-discovery—each is worthy of recognition. Creating a timeline of significant life events can be a powerful exercise, allowing you to visualize your life story and the achievements that define it.

As you map out these moments, consider how you might celebrate them. It is a simple gathering with loved ones, a quiet reflection by yourself, or a creative endeavor like writing or art. Whatever form it takes, celebrating these milestones is an opportunity to honor your time alive and the person you have become.

Organizing a celebration or gathering to commemorate your achievements can be a meaningful way to share your story with those who matter most. It does not have to be grand; even a small, intimate gathering can hold immense significance.

Consider incorporating elements that reflect your journey, such as sharing stories, displaying photographs, or creating a video montage. Such celebrations offer a chance to connect with others, to share laughter and memories, and to acknowledge the experiences that have shaped you. They are moments to pause, reflect, and appreciate our experience's richness. As you think about your milestones, remember that each one shows your resilience, growth, and unwavering spirit.

WISDOM KEEPERS: LEARNING FROM OUR ELDERS

Every community has a group of individuals whose lives are rich with the wisdom of experience. These elders, often called Wisdom Keepers, hold the keys to understanding the past and guiding the future. They serve as custodians of knowledge, preserving cultural traditions and stories that might otherwise be lost in the crazy rush of 21st-century life.

Imagine sitting with a grandparent who recounts their youth, each story a thread in the beautiful, colorful coat of your family's history. Through their words, they offer insights into times gone by, painting vivid pictures of challenges faced and overcome. This interaction is not just about sharing nostalgia; it is about passing down lessons learned and values held dear, ensuring that future generations walk with the strength and wisdom of those who came before them.

What about the story of Margaret, a beloved figure in her community known for her dedication to local environmental initiatives? Long before "sustainability" became a buzzword, Margaret advocated for practices protecting the Earth. Her wisdom, rooted in years of observation and action, inspired others to join her cause. Under her guidance, the community embarked on projects like community gardens and recycling programs, fostering a sense of stewardship among the young and the old. Margaret's influence extended beyond these practical initiatives; she taught her neighbors the importance of respecting the land and living in harmony with nature. Her legacy lives on as those she inspires carry forward her mission, planting seeds of change in their communities.

In another part of the world is Joseph, an elder passionate about traditional crafts. From weaving intricate wicker baskets to carving beautiful wooden sculptures, Joseph's hands tell stories as old as time. Recognizing the value of these skills, he has dedicated his life to teaching younger generations, ensuring that these crafts are not simply forgotten. In his workshops, Joseph shares more than techniques; he imparts the patience and perseverance that make these crafts demand. His students learn the art of creating something beautiful from raw materials, gaining skills and an appreciation for their ancestors' craftsmanship. Through his teachings, Joseph inspires a connection between the past and present, building a bridge that strengthens cultural identity and pride.

Learning from elders offers benefits that extend far beyond acquiring knowledge. Engaging with older individuals provides historical perspectives that deepen our understanding of current events. They remind us that many of the challenges we face today have been previously encountered, teaching us resilience and adaptability.

Elders offer a broad view of human experience, illuminating the cyclical nature of life and the enduring spirit that carries us through. By listening to their stories, we gain insights into the triumphs and tragedies that have shaped our ancestors, allowing us to live our lives with greater awareness and empathy.

To tap into this wellspring of wisdom, consider seeking out opportunities to connect with elders in your own life. Start by interviewing family members and asking them to share their stories and experiences. These conversations can be enriching, offering a glimpse into the lives of those who have paved the way for you.

Attend storytelling events or community gatherings where elders share their narratives, creating intergenerational learning and connection spaces. These interactions enrich your understanding and honor the contributions of those who have come before you, acknowledging their role in shaping our futures.

Engaging with Wisdom Keepers reveals the richness of our shared human heritage.

CRAFTING YOUR AGING NARRATIVE: A PERSONAL JOURNEY

Imagine sitting by a warm, cozy fire (or heater!), pen in hand, ready to draft *your* story. Crafting your aging narrative is like that —it is an opportunity to explore your life, reflect on your experiences, and shape the story you wish to tell. Drafting personal essays or memoirs can be incredibly rewarding. These writings allow you to capture the essence of your journey, the highs and lows, and *everything* in between. They serve as a bridge between your past and present, giving you clarity and insight.

You might also consider creating a vision board. This visual representation of your future aspirations can guide you toward your dreams and goals, reminding you of the possibilities ahead.

Storytelling plays a pivotal role in our personal growth. By sharing your story, you better understand who you are and what has shaped you. Participating in storytelling workshops or classes can offer a supportive environment to hone your skills and find your voice. These spaces are filled with individuals who, like you, are eager to *share* and *learn*. Your stories can resonate with others in the community or online forums, creating connections and fostering a sense of belonging.

Storytelling is empowering; it allows you to take ownership of your experiences, transforming them into narratives that reflect your truth and wisdom.

Consider engaging in practical exercises to help you articulate and shape your narrative. Developing a personal timeline of key life events can provide a structured view of your life's journey. This timeline serves as a foundation, highlighting the moments that have defined you.

Use prompts to explore themes and motifs in your life. These prompts might ask you to reflect on times of change, moments of joy, or challenges overcome. Examining these elements allows you to uncover the themes woven throughout your story, offering insights into your values and beliefs. Such exercises encourage introspection, helping you articulate your story with authenticity and depth.

Owning your story or narrative is transformative; embracing and sharing it can lead to healing and growth. Consider testimonials from individuals who have found peace through storytelling. After years of holding onto painful memories, one such person found solace by writing them down. This expression allowed them to release the weight of the past and move forward with newfound clarity.

Another story tells of a woman who, through narrative exploration, discovered a strength she never knew she had. Her story— once a source of shame became a sign of her resilience. These examples illustrate the power of storytelling to illuminate paths to healing and self-discovery.

As you craft your narrative, remember that this is *your* story. It is unique to you, shaped by *your* experiences and insights. Take the time to explore and reflect, allowing your voice to emerge.

Whether you write, create art, or share verbally, your narrative is a gift to yourself and those who care about you. By owning your story, you celebrate your life, honoring your journey and the person you have become.

CREATING A LEGACY AND LIFELONG LEARNING

One warm summer's day, I was sitting with my father on our old wooden porch, sipping lemonade, as he recounted stories of his youth. His eyes sparkled with life as he shared tales of adventures, lessons learned, and dreams pursued. As I listened, I realized these stories were more than mere memories; they were a *legacy,* tales of wisdom, courage, and love. It became clear that storytelling is an invaluable gift that preserves our history and transmits our values to the generations.

This chapter explores how *you* can leave a legacy that tells *your* story, preserving it for those who come after you.

Storytelling has always been a powerful tool for preserving history and values. Sharing your personal stories will create a legacy that extends beyond material possessions. When you write memoirs or autobiographies, you document your life experiences in a way that captures the essence of who you are. Imagine crafting a narrative that not only recounts the events of your life but also conveys the emotions, struggles, and triumphs that shaped you. This process allows you to reflect on your journey and share insights that can inspire and guide your descendants.

Creating a family history book is another beautiful way to preserve your legacy. This book becomes a living document, a connection to the people and events that preceded them. It serves as a reminder of where they came from, grounding them with a sense of identity and belonging. As they turn the pages, they will discover the values and traditions that have defined your family across generations.

In today's digital age, there are countless ways to share and preserve your stories. Consider recording video diaries or audio interviews, capturing your thoughts and reflections in your voice. These recordings can be a treasured keepsake, allowing your family to hear your laughter and wisdom long after you are gone.

Publishing stories in local newspapers or community newsletters can also be a meaningful way to share your experiences and insights with a broader audience. These publications can reach people outside your immediate family, impacting your community and leaving a legacy beyond your circle.

Organizing family storytelling evenings allows everyone to gather, share, and listen. These gatherings become a time for laughter, tears, and deepened relationships. As stories are exchanged, you create a fabric of shared experiences, bringing the family closer together. Consider making a digital archive where all family members can access these stories, ensuring they remain available for future generations.

To craft compelling and engaging narratives, consider using story prompts to spark memories and ideas. These prompts can unlock forgotten moments and lead to rich, vivid storytelling. Participating in writing workshops can also help refine your skills.

These workshops offer guidance and support, allowing you to shape your narrative with clarity and purpose.

Through storytelling, you can create a legacy that is remembered and cherished, a testament to the life you lived and the values you held dear.

Interactive Exercise: Storytelling Prompts

Take a moment to jot down a story from your life that you would like to share. Use prompts like "A lesson I learned was..." or "A time I overcame a challenge was..." to guide your reflection. As you write, focus on the emotions and insights from the experience. Consider sharing this story with a loved one or adding it to your family history book.

THE JOY OF LEARNING: NEW SKILLS AND HOBBIES

Imagine walking into a sunlit room filled with the scent of fresh paint, brushes at the ready, and a blank canvas inviting the expression of your creativity. This is the start of a new adventure where the colors of your imagination come alive. Taking up painting or drawing classes can offer a wonderful outlet for creative expression, allowing you to explore new depths of your artistic abilities. Engaging in such activities stimulates the mind, keeps the brain agile, and provides immense personal fulfillment. These newfound skills enhance creativity and bring joy and satisfaction, enriching your life unexpectedly.

Similarly, joining a cooking class can open doors to a world of flavors. Picture yourself kneading dough, chopping fresh herbs, and crafting dishes from various cuisines. It is not just about cooking but the journey of discovery. As you learn to prepare meals from diverse cultures, you expand your horizons and deepen your appreciation for food's role in connecting people across the globe.

Today, numerous resources are available to fuel your passion for learning. Online platforms like Skillshare and MasterClass offer a vast array of courses, from photography to music theory, all at your fingertips. These platforms provide flexibility, allowing you to learn at your own pace in the comfort of your home.

Additionally, local community colleges often offer workshops and classes catering to adults seeking new skills. Whether pottery, digital photography, or creative writing, there is something for everyone.

The key is to explore these resources, find what excites you, and *dive into* the learning process. With these tools, learning becomes an accessible and rewarding endeavor, regardless of age or previous experience.

Frank is a retiree who discovered the joy of music in his late sixties. He took lessons after seeing an old guitar gathering dust in his attic. What began as a casual interest quickly blossomed into quite a passion. Frank played tunes and found a sense of fulfillment and connection with others through music. Similarly, Jane took up photography after retiring from a lengthy career in teaching. She started a blog to share her photos and stories, capturing the beauty of everyday life.

Both seniors found renewed purpose and joy through these pursuits, proving that discovering new passionate interests is never too late. Their stories inspire others to explore and welcome the possibilities found in lifelong learning.

Integrating learning into your daily routine can be rewarding *and* manageable. Start by setting aside a dedicated weekly time for your new hobby or interest. This time becomes a sacred commitment to yourself, an appointment for personal growth. Whether it is an hour spent painting or a morning devoted to writing, these moments add up, creating a life of progress and achievement.

Creating a learning plan with specific goals and milestones can also help keep you motivated and focused. Write down what you hope to achieve in the coming weeks or months. Set attainable targets, such as completing a certain number of lessons or producing a finished work.

As you embark on this journey of learning and discovery, remember that the *process* is as valuable as the *result*. Allow yourself to explore, experiment, and make mistakes! Each step forward is a step toward growth, bringing a sense of achievement and satisfaction. Embrace the joy of learning; knowing each new skill or hobby enriches your life and adds to your legacy.

Whether painting, cooking, or playing an instrument, these activities will become a part of who you are, reflecting your passions and curiosities.

EMBRACING CHANGE: ADAPTING AND THRIVING

Change is a constant companion in our lives, often becoming unbidden and unsettling but offering pathways to growth and new opportunities. Embracing change is crucial for personal development, allowing us to explore uncharted territories and expand our horizons.

Consider the way technology has transformed our personal and professional lives. Not so long ago, using smartphones and the internet seemed impossible to many. Yet, by taking small steps, such as learning to send an email or video call to a loved one, many have harnessed these tools to stay connected and engaged in a rapidly evolving world. These adaptations have connected us globally and allowed for continued learning and interaction, enriching our lives in countless ways.

Relocating to a new place can be another formidable change that, while challenging, often leads to personal growth and fulfillment. Imagine moving to a different city (or even country), surrounded by unfamiliar faces and customs. The initial discomfort can give way to a thriving new existence, as seen in the stories of those who have made such moves.

People often find that relocating forces them to step outside their comfort zones, fostering resilience and adaptability. New environments offer fresh perspectives and opportunities to learn about diverse cultures, traditions, and ways of life. This openness can lead to personal enrichment, more profound empathy, and a broader world understanding.

Developing adaptability requires a willingness to remain open to new experiences and perspectives. It means stepping outside familiar routines and engaging in activities that challenge preconceived notions. Whether trying a new hobby, attending events with diverse groups, or traveling to unfamiliar places, these experiences can broaden your outlook and enhance your adaptability.

Practicing flexibility in everyday situations, such as trying different foods or altering daily routines, can also build resilience. By welcoming the unknown, you develop a mindset that is open to change and *eager* for it, ready to see what each new experience might bring!

A positive mindset is pivotal in navigating such change with grace and resilience. Maintaining a hopeful outlook can ease transitions and make adapting to new circumstances less frightening. Using affirmations can help build confidence, reminding you of your strength and capability to face whatever comes your way. Phrases like "I am adaptable and resilient" or "Change brings new opportunities" reinforce a positive attitude, making challenges feel more like productive stepping stones than obstacles.

Journaling can also be a powerful tool for processing thoughts and emotions during times of transition. Writing down your feelings allows you to reflect on them more objectively, helping you identify patterns and work through any discomfort or uncertainty you may feel.

Consider the story of an elder who found a new purpose by transitioning into a *completely* different career after retirement. A former accountant, she discovered a passion for teaching and began tutoring math at a local community center. This shift not only enriched her life but also had a profound impact on the students she mentored. Her ability to adapt to a new role brought her joy and a sense of fulfillment she had not anticipated.

Similarly, becoming a grandparent can be another profound life change. While it may initially seem overwhelming, many find it brings unexpected happiness and deepens family bonds.

Change can be scary, but it also holds the potential for transformation and growth. You will live through life's transitions with confidence and resilience by embracing change, cultivating adaptability, and maintaining a positive outlook.

PLANNING FOR THE FUTURE: A LEGACY OF LOVE

Thoughtful planning for the future ensures that your values and love are reflected in the legacy you leave behind. It involves more than distributing your assets; it is about ensuring your life's work and values *continue to inspire* long after you are gone.

Creating a will or trust is a fundamental step in this process. These documents outline your wishes clearly, providing guidance and security for your loved ones. A well-constructed will or trust can prevent potential disputes and ensure that your assets are distributed according to your desires. This planning brings peace of mind, knowing that your intentions are documented and will be honored.

Writing letters to family members is another heartfelt way to express love and offer guidance. These letters provide an individualized touch that legal documents cannot. They allow you to share wisdom, hopes, and dreams with your loved ones, creating a lasting connection.

Imagine a grandchild reading your words years from now, feeling your presence and love through the lines you wrote. These letters can become cherished keepsakes, offering comfort and inspiration throughout the lives of your family members. They remind them of your values and the lessons you learned, guiding them as they travel their paths.

Involving your family in legacy planning can strengthen bonds and ensure your values are understood and upheld. Hosting family meetings to discuss your legacy goals and values creates a collaborative environment where everyone can contribute and feel included. These discussions can enlighten, revealing shared values and aspirations that can guide the family's future. Collaborating on family projects or initiatives that reflect these values can further reinforce the legacy you wish to leave.

Setting up scholarships or charitable funds in your name can extend your influence and support causes you hold dear. These acts of giving continue your legacy, promoting values of kindness and generosity. Establishing family traditions that endure over time reinforces the love and values you wish to pass down.

Traditions like annual gatherings or shared rituals can create lasting memories and strengthen familial bonds, offering a sense of continuity and belonging.

Working with financial advisors who can ensure that your resources align with your legacy goals helps create a comprehensive legacy plan. These professionals can guide you through the complexities of legacy planning, providing advice and support to make informed decisions. Legacy planning tools and templates can help capture your wishes and values, streamlining the process and ensuring nothing is overlooked. Organizing and documenting your intentions will create a roadmap that guides your loved ones and honors your life's work.

As you reflect on the legacy you want to leave, consider the values and love that have defined your life. Use this reflection to guide your planning, ensuring that your legacy represents who you are and what you stand for. Take the opportunity to create something lasting and meaningful, knowing that your love and values will *continue* to inspire and guide those you leave behind.

CONCLUSION

As we reach the end of this book, I invite you to reflect on the vision that inspired this writing: to empower you to embrace aging as a period of vitality and wisdom.

We set out to shift perceptions, replacing fear and uncertainty with joy and fulfillment. Aging is not merely about living with time; it is a transformative experience with opportunities for growth, learning, and connection!

Throughout these pages, we have explored essential themes contributing to a fulfilling life as we age. We delved into maintaining physical vitality through tailored exercises and nutrition, emphasizing how cultivating a healthy body supports longevity. We discussed the importance of mental sharpness and cognitive health, highlighting techniques to keep your mind engaged and resilient. Emotional well-being emerged as a cornerstone, reminding us that nurturing our inner world will foster our resilience and happiness.

Social connections and community engagement enrich our lives, providing support and companionship. We also examined financial security, offering peace of mind and independence strategies. Spiritual growth and cultural perspectives give a broader understanding of aging, encouraging you to participate in diverse practices that enrich your spirit. Each theme builds upon the others, creating a comprehensive approach to living your *best* years.

Reflect on the key takeaways from each chapter. Consistent movement and mindful nutrition can enhance physical vitality. Cognitive exercises, lifelong learning, and mindfulness practices benefit the mind. Emotional intelligence, gratitude, and resilience are tools for gracefully facing life's challenges. Building strong social networks and engaging with your community can bring joy and purpose. Financial planning ensures security, while spiritual and cultural practices offer more profound meaning and connection.

Remember the success stories we shared—stories of individuals who welcomed change and found fulfillment in unexpected places. These narratives serve as a testament to the power of perspective. People like Susan, Jack, and Mary showed us that pursuing new dreams is never too late.

As you move forward, let this book be a guide and companion. I continue to learn and grow. Seek out new experiences and find knowledge to enrich your journey. Stay curious and open-minded. *Your* story is *still* being written, and each day is an opportunity to add a new chapter!

Now, I heartily encourage you to take specific steps toward applying the insights and strategies shared in this book. Set personal goals for your health, nurture your relationships, secure your finances, and explore your spiritual path. Engage with your community and share your stories. Inspire others by living *your* truth and supporting collective growth.

As we conclude, stride onto this stage of your life with confidence and an open heart. Aging offers empowerment, joy, and fulfillment. It is quite a privilege to grow older to witness the world through the lens of accumulated wisdom. Approach these years with courage and enthusiasm, ready to make the most of your *best* years!

I invite you to contact me through social media or my website. Let us continue this conversation, supporting one another as we age and feeling empowered.

We can create a community of strength, wisdom, and joy.

BE AN INSPIRATION!

I hope you see the incredible, true potential of the later stage of life ahead of you now and feel ready to embrace it with *strength* and *positivity*.

Take a moment now to help others do the same.

By sharing your honest opinion of this book and how it has changed your perspective, you will inspire new readers to improve their view of aging and embrace their later years with positivity and enthusiasm.

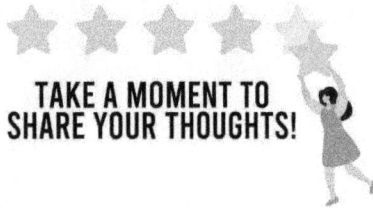

TAKE A MOMENT TO SHARE YOUR THOUGHTS!

Thank you so much for your support.

I wish you many happy and vibrant years ahead!

REFERENCES

U.S. Department of Health and Human Services. (2018). Physical Activity Guidelines for Americans (2nd ed.). https://health.gov/sites/default/files/2019-09/Physical_Activity_Guidelines_2nd_edition.pdf

Gómez-Pinilla, F. (2008). Brain foods: The effects of nutrients on brain function. *Nature Reviews Neuroscience, 9*(7), 568-578. https://doi.org/10.1038/nrn2421

Emmons, R. A., & McCullough, M. E. (2003). Counting blessings versus burdens: An experimental investigation of gratitude and subjective well-being in daily life. *Journal of Personality and Social Psychology, 84*(2), 377-389. https://doi.org/10.1037/0022-3514.84.2.377

Shah, A. A., & Wilson, R. S. (2020). The impact of social interactions on cognitive flexibility in aging adults. *Journal of Geriatric Psychiatry and Neurology, 33*(5), 290-298. https://doi.org/10.1177/0891988719888491

Smith, A., & Anderson, M. (2018). *Mobile technology and its impact on social well-being: Keeping connected to family and healthcare resources.* Pew Research Center. https://www.pewresearch.org/internet/2018/11/15/mobile-technology-and-its-impact-on-social-well-being

Ramsey Solutions. (n.d.). EveryDollar budgeting app: A tool for informed spending decisions. https://www.ramseysolutions.com/ever-dollar

YNAB. (n.d.). You Need a Budget (YNAB): Take control of your money. https://www.youneedabudget.com/

National Council on Aging. (2023). NCOA partners with AT&T to boost the digital skills of older adults. https://www.ncoa.org/article/national-council-on-aging-partners-with-att-to-boost-tech-skills-of-older-adults

"10 Quotes About the Beauty of Aging". (2022) Home Instead. Last modified January 14, 2022. https://www.homeinstead.com/location/529/news-and-media/10-quotes-about-the-beauty-of-aging/.

National Institutes of Health. (n.d.). Growth mindset predicts cognitive gains in an older adult. https://www.ncbi.nlm.nih.gov/pmc/articles/PMC10052424/

The Gerontologist. (2023). What does it mean to age successfully?: Multinational study. https://academic.oup.com/gerontologist/article/64/10/gnae102/7731211

Senior Lifestyle. (n.d.). Why lifelong learning is important for seniors. https://www.seniorlifestyle.com/resources/blog/lifelong-learning-for-seniors/

Harvard T.H. Chan School of Public Health. (n.d.). Positive attitude about aging could boost health. https://www.hsph.harvard.edu/news/hsph-in-the-news/positive-attitude-about-aging-could-boost-health/

Centers for Disease Control and Prevention (CDC). (n.d.). Physical activity benefits for adults 65 or older. https://www.cdc.gov/physical-activity-basics/health-benefits/older-adults.html

National Council on Aging. (n.d.). The 8 best superfoods for seniors. https://www.ncoa.org/article/the-8-best-superfoods-for-seniors/

Mayo Clinic. (n.d.). Exercising with arthritis: Improve your joint pain and stiffness. https://www.mayoclinic.org/diseases-conditions/arthritis/in-depth/arthritis/art-20047971

National Institutes of Health. (n.d.). Effectiveness of Tai Chi for health promotion of older adults. https://www.ncbi.nlm.nih.gov/pmc/articles/PMC9644143/

National Institutes of Health. (n.d.). Effects of omega-3 polyunsaturated fatty acids on brain health in older adults. https://pmc.ncbi.nlm.nih.gov/articles/PMC9641984/

National Institutes of Health. (n.d.). Mindfulness-based interventions for older adults. https://www.ncbi.nlm.nih.gov/pmc/articles/PMC4868399/

National Institutes of Health. (n.d.). Preventive strategies for cognitive decline and dementia. https://www.ncbi.nlm.nih.gov/pmc/articles/PMC10046723/

National Institutes of Health. (n.d.). Antioxidant intervention to improve cognition in the aging brain. https://www.ncbi.nlm.nih.gov/pmc/articles/PMC9778814/

Atlas Senior Living. (n.d.). Emotional intelligence: Develop as the key to healthy aging. https://atlasseniorliving.com/blog/emotional-intelligence-develop-as-the-key-to-healthy-aging/

National Institutes of Health. (n.d.). The effects of gratitude interventions: A systematic review. https://www.ncbi.nlm.nih.gov/pmc/articles/PMC10393216/

The Encore Project. (n.d.). The power of resilience: Stories from senior lives. https://theencoreproject.org/inspiration-personal-growth/the-power-of-resilience-stories-from-senior-lives/

National Institutes of Health. (n.d.). Purpose in life in older adults: A systematic review. https://www.ncbi.nlm.nih.gov/pmc/articles/PMC9141815/

Mayo Clinic. (n.d.). A surprising key to healthy aging: Strong social connections. https://mcpress.mayoclinic.org/healthy-aging/a-surprising-key-to-healthy-aging-strong-social-connections/

National Institutes of Health. (n.d.). The use of digital technology for social well-being reduces isolation among older adults. https://www.ncbi.nlm.nih.gov/pmc/articles/PMC8733322/

BMC Public Health. (2021). Community participation of community-dwelling older adults. https://bmcpublichealth.biomedcentral.com/articles/10.1186/s12889-021-10592-4

Forbes. (n.d.). 11 meaningful ways older adults can volunteer right now. https://www.forbes.com/health/healthy-aging/volunteer-opportunities-for-older-adults/

Senior Living. (n.d.). Best budgeting for seniors in 2024. https://www.seniorliving.org/finance/budgeting-apps/

Covenant Wealth Advisors. (n.d.). Where to invest emergency funds in retirement. https://www.covenantwealthadvisors.com/post/where-to-invest-emergency-funds-in-retirement

T. Rowe Price. (n.d.). Six steps to achieve financial independence and retire early. https://www.troweprice.com/personal-investing/resources/insights/6-steps-to-achieve-financial-independence-and-retire-early.html

AARP. (n.d.). Public benefits – Senior assistance. https://www.aarp.org/aarp-foundation/our-work/income/public-benefits-guide-senior-assistance/

Mindworks. (n.d.). Best meditation techniques for seniors. https://mindworks.org/blog/best-meditation-techniques-seniors/

National Institutes of Health. (n.d.). Mindfulness-based interventions for older adults. https://www.ncbi.nlm.nih.gov/pmc/articles/PMC4868399/

Merck Manuals. (n.d.). Religion and spirituality in older adults. https://www.merckmanuals.com/professional/geriatrics/social-issues-in-older-adults/religion-and-spirituality-in-older-adults

Psychology Today. (2023, October). The benefits of a life review exercise long before death. https://www.psychologytoday.com/us/blog/4000-mondays/202310/the-benefits-of-a-life-review-exercise-long-before-death

U.S. Pain Foundation. (n.d.). Holistic approaches to chronic pain. https://uspainfoundation.org/blog/holistic-approaches-to-chronic-pain/

Healthline. (n.d.). 9 home remedies backed by science. https://www.healthline.com/health/home-remedies

HR Cloud. (n.d.). How to build a well-connected healthcare team. https://www.hrcloud.com/blog/how-to-build-a-well-connected-healthcare-team

A Place for Mom. (n.d.). Medication management for seniors: Tips from a doctor. https://www.aplaceformom.com/caregiver-resources/articles/medication-management

National Council on Aging. (n.d.). New program helps older adults with tech skills. https://www.ncoa.org/article/national-council-on-aging-partners-with-att-to-boost-tech-skills-of-older-adults/

A Place for Mom. (n.d.). Best apps for seniors in 2024: Fun, health, and convenience. https://www.aplaceformom.com/caregiver-resources/articles/best-apps-for-seniors

ConnectSafely. (n.d.). The senior's guide to online safety. https://connectsafely.org/seniors-guide-to-online-safety/

Pennsylvania State University. (n.d.). Using technology to connect generations. https://aese.psu.edu/outreach/intergenerational/program-areas/technology

National Institutes of Health. (n.d.). Blue Zones: Lessons from the world's longest-lived. https://pmc.ncbi.nlm.nih.gov/articles/PMC6125071/

National Institutes of Health. (n.d.). Ayurveda and the science of aging. https://www.ncbi.nlm.nih.gov/pmc/articles/PMC6148064/

Gueye, R. (n.d.). The vital role of elders in African communities. https://rabygueye.medium.com/the-vital-role-of-elders-in-african-communities-0e72422076cb

Charles Sturt University. (n.d.). Ubuntu-informed care for the elderly: Towards a holistic care approach. https://researchoutput.csu.edu.au/en/publications/ubuntu-informed-care-for-the-elderly-towards-a-holistic-care-for

Daily Plate of Crazy. (2017, January 15). Success stories later in life: Over 50, over 60, overcoming losses. https://dailyplateofcrazy.com/2017/01/15/success-stories-later-in-life-over-50-over-60-overcoming-losses/

National Institutes of Health. (n.d.). Resilience and successful aging. https://www.ncbi.nlm.nih.gov/pmc/articles/PMC9209635/

Abiding Home Care. (n.d.). Celebrating life's milestones: Meaningful ways to honor seniors on special occasions. https://abidinghc.com/celebrating-lifes-milestones-meaningful-ways-to-honor-seniors-on-special-occasions/

Wisdom Keepers. (n.d.). Reigniting the ancient ways. https://www.wisdomkeepers.earth/

Brown Brothers Harriman. (n.d.). Storytelling in wealth and legacy: Preserving values across generations. https://www.bbh.com/us/en/insights/capital-partners-insights/storytelling-in-wealth-and-legacy.html

United Nations Educational, Scientific and Cultural Organization (UNESCO). (n.d.). The benefits of lifelong learning for older adults. https://www.uil.unesco.org/en/thematic-studies-benefits-lifelong-learning-older-adults

National Institutes of Health. (n.d.). Adapting to aging: Older people talk about their use of technology. https://www.ncbi.nlm.nih.gov/pmc/articles/PMC5927091/

Thrivent Financial. (n.d.). What do you need to know about legacy planning, and how do you get started? What you need to know about legacy planning & how to get started

www.ingramcontent.com/pod-product-compliance
Lightning Source LLC
Chambersburg PA
CBHW022059020426
42335CB00012B/755